Health Informatics
(formerly Computers in Health Care)

Kathryn J. Hannah   Marion J. Ball
Series Editors

For other titles published in this series, go to
www.springer.com/series/1114

Nancy B. Finn • William F. Bria

Digital Communication in Medical Practice

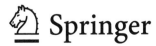 Springer

Nancy B. Finn
Communication Resources
Needham, MA
USA

William F. Bria
Shriners Hospitals for Children
2900 Rocky Point Drive
Tampa, FL
USA

ISBN 978-1-84882-354-9   e-ISBN 978-1-84882-355-6
DOI: 10.1007/978-1-84882-355-6

British Library Cataloguing in Publication Data

Library of Congress Control Number: 2008944093

Printed on acid-free paper

Springer London is part of Springer Science + Business Media (www.springer.com)

To our children and grandchildren who are the future: Jeffrey, Glenn, Alex, Marc, David, Ivy, Gefen and Sydney Finn, Bill and James Bria

Foreword

Enabling the Complexity of Communication in Health Care

The cost, quality, safety, and access problems of healthcare are well known. These problems are based in and exacerbated by the complexity of healthcare. The knowledge domain of medicine is vast and evolves rapidly. Patients and providers have an asymmetry of knowledge and experience. Patients with complex acute problems and multiple chronic disease will be seen by many providers within a short period of time and will be undergoing several, parallel treatments. The delivery system is highly fragmented and dominated by small physician groups and hospitals. Reimbursement mechanisms do not sufficiently reward care coordination and care that is safe, efficient, and uses the best medical evidence. Managed care contract provisions can fill volumes.

Over the years we have learned that information technology can be applied to help address many of the challenges faced by healthcare. We have also learned that these gains are not an automatic result of application implementation. Systems design must be thoughtful. Care processes and workflow must be skillfully accommodated and changed. Training must be provided on an ongoing basis. Means must exist for the provider to cover the initial and ongoing costs of the technology. However, when all of these parallel efforts are carried out, there is a large body of evidence that care improvement can be significant.

Stepping back from these experiences, one realizes the fundamental contribution of information technology – it enables complexity. Our financial assets are much more complex than those of our grandparents; savings accounts have been replaced by retirement plans and mutual funds that automatically shift assets based on a person's risk tolerance. Handwritten flight manifests have been replaced by the ability of an individual to book air travel involving multiple stops and carriers. Weather forecasting based on seasonal expectations and reports from adjacent states has been replaced by sophisticated models. Complex activities such as sending a satellite to Jupiter, noninvasively observing metabolism in the brain and simulating the interactions between proteins would not be possible without information technology.

Information technology can be applied to enable the complexity in healthcare. Clinical decision support and clinical documentation applications can assist the provider in keeping up with medical evidence. Results management systems can highlight the patient data that deserves the most attention. Interoperable electronic health records can support the coordination of multiple providers taking care of an elderly patient. Telemedicine can assist patients and providers in joint management of chronic disease.

Decades old methods of paper and telephone are not sufficiently potent to be effective tools in managing today's complex healthcare. As a result, the health care system breaks – repeatedly and with often dire consequences.

Communication is one of the most essential processes in healthcare. It is also one of the most complex. Communication occurs between many participants – patients and their provider(s), primary care providers and specialists, professional societies and practitioners, patients and other patients, and providers and health insurance companies. The "language" used in the communication is often arcane, multifaceted, and incomplete. Leveraging information technology to enable the complex process of communication in healthcare will enable a healthcare system that not only breaks less often but is more efficient, effective, and safe.

Nancy Finn and Bill Bria have done a superb job of addressing the challenge of communication in healthcare using information technology. Digital Communication in Medical Practice provides an insightful, practical, thorough, and highly readable discussion of the roles that information technology can play in improving the ability of the physician to communicate with their patients and other providers. The authors provide a holistic view that integrates a review of the technology with the necessary parallel activities such as process change and training.

Over the course of the last decade, there has been explosive innovation in communications technologies: the Internet, electronic health record, and personal health records, the cell phone, electronic mail, remote monitoring technologies. All of these technologies have witnessed significant increases in their capabilities and a rapidly maturing understanding of how to apply them. These innovations offer us new opportunities to improve care.

Information technology can enable us to master the complexity of communication in healthcare. This mastery will allow us to craft the healthcare delivery system that our patients and providers deserve. Digital Communication in Medical Practice moves us significantly toward that goal.

John Glaser, PhD
Vice President and CIO
Partners Healthcare

Series Preface

This series is directed to Healthcare professionals who are leading the transformation of health care by using information and knowledge. Historically, the series was launched in 1988 as Computers in Health Care, to offer a broad range of titles: some addressed to specific professions such as nursing, medicine, and health administration; others to special areas of practice such as trauma and radiology; still other books in the series focused on interdisciplinary issues, such as the computer-based patient record, electronic health records, and networked Healthcare systems. Renamed Health Informatics in 1998 to reflect the rapid evolution in the discipline known as health Informatics, the series continued to add titles that contribute to the evolution of the field. In the series, eminent experts, serving as editors or authors, offer their accounts of innovations in health Informatics. Increasingly, these accounts go beyond hardware and software to address the role of information in influencing the transformation of Healthcare delivery systems around the world. The series also increasingly focused on the users of the information and systems: the organizational, behavioral, and societal changes that accompany the diffusion of information technology in health services environments.

Developments in healthcare delivery are constant; most recently developments in proteomics and genomics are increasingly becoming relevant to clinical decision making and emerging standards of care. The data resources emerging from molecular biology are beyond the capacity of the human brain to integrate and beyond the scope of paper-based decision trees. Thus, bioinformatics has emerged as a new field in health informatics to support emerging and ongoing developments in molecular biology. Translational informatics supports acceleration, from bench to bedside, i.e., the appropriate use of molecular biology research findings and bioinformatics in clinical care of patients.

At the same time, further continual evolution of the field of Health informatics is reflected in the introduction of concepts at the macro or health systems delivery level with major national initiatives related to electronic health records (EHR), data standards, and public health informatics such as the Healthcare Information Technology Standards Panel (HITSP) in the United States, Canada Health Infoway, NHS Connecting for Health in the UK.

We have consciously retained the series title Health Informatics as the single umbrella term that encompasses both the microscopic elements of bioinformatics and the macroscopic aspects of large national health information systems. Ongoing changes to both the micro and macro perspectives on health informatics will continue to shape health services in the twenty-first century. By making full and creative use of the technology to tame data and to transform information, health Informatics will foster the development and use of new knowledge in health care. As coeditors, we pledge to support our professional colleagues and the series readers as they share advances in the emerging and exciting field of Health Informatics.

Kathryn J. Hannah
Marion J. Ball

Acknowledgments

We are pleased to acknowledge the assistance of many individuals who contributed their time, thoughts, and expertise to this book because they believe in health information technology as a way to provide safer, better quality healthcare to patients throughout the world.

We owe a special thanks to Dr. Dan Teres, whose mentoring and insightful review comments kept this book on track. Several individuals devoted significant time and effort to help us understand the impact of various health information technologies and their impact. They include Dr. Joseph Kvedor from the Center for Connected Health whose invaluable assistance provided us with the appropriate focus on telemedicine; Dr. Danny Sands, an evangelist and a pioneer in the use of electronic health records, email, and patient portals; Susanna Fox and the PEW Institute whose cutting edge research provides invaluable insights in how people use the Internet; John Glaser who devoted enormous time and effort guiding us through some of the technical material; Dena Puskin who early on provided connections to key thought leaders in Health IT; Michele Garvin Esq. of Ropes and Gray LLP who guided us through the difficult legal issues of privacy. We owe a special thanks to Missy Goldberg who meticulously worked with the authors to proofread the content and to Tania Helhoski of Bird Design who assisted with graphics. We thank the editors at Springer Publishing. We recognize the following healthcare professionals who bought into the idea for this book and provided value added materials and thoughts:

Tom Abrams, Director Division of Drug Marketing, Advertising, and Communications (DDMAC), Food and Drug Administration.

Holt Anderson, Executive Director, North Carolina Health Information and Communications Alliance.

John Blair, MD, President & CEO, Taconic IPA.

William Braithwaite, MD, PhD, FACMI Health Information Policy Advisor.

Claire Broome, MD, Director Integrated Health Information Systems, Centers for Disease Control and Prevention.

Todd Brown, MHP, RPh, Associate Clinical Specialist and Vice Chair, Department of Pharmacy Practice School of Pharmacy, Northeastern University.

Gary Christopherson, MD, Senior Advisor; Undersecretary for Health, Veterans Administration Senior Fellow, Institute of Medicine.

Homer L. Chin, MD, Medical Director, Clinical Information Systems, Kaiser Permanente.

David Classen, MD, Vice President, First Consulting Group.

Jeffrey Cooper, PhD, Director of Biomedical Engineering, Partners Healthcare, Boston, MA.

Robert Cox, MD, Director Hays Medical Center, Hays Kansas.

Tom Delbanco, MD, Primary Care Medicine, Beth Israel Deaconess Medical Center, Boston, MA.

Suzanne Delbanco, PhD, The Leapfrog Group.

Henry DePhillips, MD, Chief Medical Officer, Medem.

George Demetri, MD, Director of Center for Sarcoma and Bone Oncology, Dana Farber Cancer Institute, Associate Professor of Medicine Harvard Medical School.

Don E. Detmer, MD, MA, President and CEO, American Medical Informatics Association.

Tom Ferguson, MD, doctortom.com, pioneer in health informatics (deceased).

Ross D. Fletcher, MD, Chief of Staff VA Medical Center, Washington, DC.

Mark Foster, MD, Vice Chairman, Taconic IPA Inc., Chairman, THINC RHIO.

Susannah Fox, Pew Internet & American Life Project.

Charles Ganley, MD, Director, Division of Over-the-Counter Drug Products.

Michele M. Garvin, Esq. Partner, Health Care Group, Ropes & Gray LLP.

John Glaser, Vice President and CIO Partners Healthcare.

JanLori Goldman, Columbia Health Privacy Project.

John Halamka, MD, MS, Chief Information Officer, Caregroup Health System, Chief Information Officer, Harvard Medical School.

Claus Hamann, MD, MS, FRCP(C), Geriatric Primary Care Massachusetts General Hospital.

Matthew R. Handley, MD, Family Practice, Group Health Cooperative, Seattle, WA.

Carol Holquist, RPh, Director, Division of Medication Errors and Technology Support, FDA, Washington, DC.

Joel Kahn, MD, President, WorldCare Global Health Plan.

Charles M. Kilo, MD, MPH, Greenfield Health, Portland, OR.

Joseph C. Kvedor, MD, Director, Center for Connected Health, Partners Healthcare.

Howard M. Landa, MD, Kaiser Permanente Department of Pediatric Urology.

Thomas F. Landholt, MD, Family Practice, Springfield, MO.

David J. Lansky, PhD, Senior Advisor on Health Policy.

Mark Leavitt, MD, PhD, Chairman of the Certification Commission for Healthcare, Information Technology (CCHIT).

Eric Liederman, MD, MPH, Director of Medical Informatics, Kaiser Permanante UC Davis, Health Systems.

Steven R. Levisohn, MD, Primary Care, Massachusetts General Hospital, Boston, MA.

Janet Marchibroda, CEO and Founder, eHealth Initiative.

Robert J. Mandel, MD, MBA, eHealth Program, Blue Cross Blue Shield, Massachusetts.

David Nash, MD, MBA, Professor and Chairman of Health Policy, Thomas Jefferson University, Jefferson Medical College, Philadelphia, PA.

Larry Nathanson, MD, Director, Emergency Medicine Informatics, Beth Israel Deaconess Medical Center, Boston, MA.

Marc Overhage, MD, President and CEO of the Indiana Health Information Exchange.

Dena Puskin, ScD, Director, Federal Office for the Advancement of Telehealth, U.S. Department of Health and Human Services.

Brian Rosenfeld, MD, Founder VISICU Inc.

Steve Ross, MD, U Colorado Health Science Center, U Colorado Hospital.

Jay H. Sanders, MD, President and CEO of The Global Telemedicine Group, Professor of Medicine at Johns Hopkins University School of Medicine.

Danny Sands, MD, Assistant Clinical Professor of Medicine at Harvard Medical School and Senior Medical Informatics Director for Cisco Systems Inc.

Joseph Scherger, MD, MPH, Professor of Clinical Family and Preventive Medicine at the University of California, San Diego School of Medicine.

Steve Schneider, MD, CMO, Healthwise.

Hasan Sharif, MD, COO, CMO, WorldCare.

Warner Slack, MD, Department of Neurology, Beth Israel Deaconess Medical Center, Boston, MA, Pioneer Informatics.

Paul Tang, MD, MS, Vice President and Chief Medical Information Officer, Palo Alto Medical Foundation (PAMF), Stanford, CA.

Lisa Vetter, Telemedicine Specialist, St. Alexius Medical Center, North Dakota.

Jonathan S. Wald, MD, MPH, Associate Director of the Clinical Informatics, Research and Development (CIRD) Group, Partners Healthcare.

Andy Wiesenthal, MD, Associate Executive Director for Clinical Information Support, The Permanente Federation.

David Williams Principal, MedPharma Partners LLC.

Contents

Introduction
A Visit to the Doctor: Three Scenarios

Scenario #1

Dr. Jennifer Hathaway, a primary care physician in a suburb of Chicago starts her day with 25 files piled on her desk, representing the 25 patients that she will see in the next eight hours. Her first patient is Eleanor, a healthy 45-year-old woman, who works as a software engineer. Eleanor is waiting for the doctor in the examining room after Dr. Smith's medical assistant has taken her vitals and weight, draws blood and does an EKG, which she attaches to Eleanor's chart. Eleanor has also filled in an update form that has been placed at the front of her chart.

Dr. Hathaway enters the examining room, carrying Eleanor's file. She gives it a quick glance noting Eleanor's weight, blood pressure, and a note about headaches. She greets Eleanor, shakes her hand and warmly welcomes her back for her annual visit, observing stress in Eleanor's face and a slight tremor in the handshake. Eleanor has been a patient for the past 10 years, and they banter back and forth about her general health and her family. While examining Eleanor, Dr. Hathaway asks about any new issues or changes, as she has not had time to read the update form that Eleanor filled out. When she is finished Dr. Hathaway suggests that Eleanor get dressed, and meet her in her office.

While she is waiting for Eleanor, Dr. Hathaway quickly reads her update form and skims through her record, seeking information from the last visit. As they talk Dr. Hathaway takes copious notes in longhand. She tells Eleanor that her blood pressure is quite high compared to a year ago and suggests that could be the cause of her headaches. She recommends that Eleanor start a hypertension medication and have a stress test. She writes out prescriptions and slips for lab work, which she hands to Eleanor, reassuring her that there is nothing to worry about.

After the visit, Dr. Hathaway collects and reviews all of Eleanor's labs and test results and within a couple of weeks she sends Eleanor a note indicating that her stress test and other blood work is normal, but her cholesterol is high. She encloses a prescription for a cholesterol medication and tells Eleanor to call if she has questions.

Unfortunately, the cholesterol medication makes Eleanor dizzy so she calls the office the next day and leaves a message. Dr. Hathaway calls her back, but Eleanor is not there. It takes three days and two more rounds of telephone calls before the doctor and

N.B. Finn and W.F. Bria, *Digital Communication in Medical Practice*,
DOI: 10.1007/978-1-84882-355-6_1, © Springer-Verlag London Limited 2009

Eleanor connect. Dr. Hathaway tells Eleanor to immediately stop what she is taking and indicates that she will call a new drug into the pharmacy. There is no further communication between Dr. Hathaway and Eleanor until her next visit six months later.

Scenario #2

Dr. James Thatcher, who practices general medicine in a community just outside Atlanta, GA, is proud of the fact that, after much time, expense, and energy, his office has installed a new computer system with electronic records for all of his patients, a medications database, and e-prescribing capability. Dr. Thatcher and his staff spent a weekend in training to help them use and understand the new computer system.

When his patient Dan, a retired 80-year-old contractor with asthma and high blood pressure, comes in for his six-month visit, he gives his medical card to an office attendant, who looks up his patient record on the computer and confirms his identity and birth date. Dan is still asked to fill out a paper update form that he struggles with as he tries to remember all of the dosages for his medications and recall his family medical history.

As Dan enters the exam room, Dr. Thatcher is at the computer reviewing his electronic medical record (EMR). They talk for a few minutes and after examining Dan, the doctor notes the start of a bronchial infection. While Dan waits, Dr. Thatcher searches his new medication database to find the right antibiotic to treat Dan's bronchitis. The computer returns with a list of three medications that would be appropriate, and flags one of the medications that Dan's health plan will not accept. The doctor makes his choice and electronically transmits the prescription to Dan's local pharmacy where the computer prints a concise set of instructions including a warning on potential side effects and directions about how Dan should take the drug.

Once again Dr. Thatcher turns his attention to Dan and together they review Dan's electronic medical record on the computer and discuss some of the most recent entries. Dr Thatcher prints a list of web links where Dan can find information about the new prescription and other medical issues. Dan's prescription is waiting when he arrives at the pharmacy on his way home.

Scenario #3

Anne Downes is a primary care physician in Minnesota, who has always been intrigued with technology and early on adopted an electronic medical record as her way of keeping patient charts. But Anne is not satisfied with having a static set of patient records online. She believes in using technology tools for patient communication and seamless interaction between her prescribing systems, billing systems, health insurance providers and the hospital where she has admitting privileges.

When Dr. Downes' patients are scheduled for an office visit, they must do some of the preparatory work ahead so that she is able to devote 100 percent of her focus and time to talking, examining, and listening to her patients.

Donna is a 57-year-old teacher with chronic diabetes and arthritis. Donna sees Dr. Downes every four months. Ten days before her scheduled visit, Donna receives an email from Dr. Downes with a link to the portal that Dr. Downes shares with her patients, reminding Donna to go to her private section of the portal and enter her most recent blood sugar readings from her glucometer. The readings are automatically graphed by the computer and available for Dr. Downes to review before the visit.

When Donna arrives at Dr. Downe's office, she goes directly to a computer terminal where she scans her medical card. This automatically notifies the office staff and Dr. Downes that she has arrived, and brings up Donna's electronic health record. Earlier in the day, an automated computer program sent a checklist of all the patients scheduled to Dr. Downe's PDA. From that device she is able to access Donna's record and determine the agenda for their visit.

When she arrives, Donna is escorted to an examining room where a nurse takes her blood pressure, weight, and other vitals and keys the information directly into Donna's health record on the computer. She leaves that screen visible for Dr. Downes. Having already seen Donna's record and her latest entries on her PDA, Dr. Downes is able to look very quickly at the computer screen to assess Donna's condition. As a result, during the 15 minutes allotted to the visit, Dr. Downes is able to focus completely on Donna and concentrate on their discussion without the distraction of having to write notes or look up information. Donna explains that she has been experiencing pain in her shoulders and tingling down her arms. Dr. Downes recommends that she should see a neurologist who will run some tests. She also prescribes a new diabetes medication.

At the conclusion of the visit, Dr. Downes takes a few minutes to send a prescription directly from her computer to the pharmacy; an email to a neurologist with a note about Donna's symptoms; and to post links to Donna's patient portal site. The computer automatically transfers all the information about the prescription, the symptoms, and the referral to the neurologist to Donna's electronic health record. Dr. Downes reminds Donna that if she has any questions she can send her an email. She feels satisfied that although her time with her patient is limited, these digital tools provide her with information and communication that enables a comprehensive, unrushed visit.

As she leaves the office, Donna goes to a kiosk where a computer survey is on the screen that asks questions about Donna's satisfaction with the visit. With this information Dr. Downes is able to make adjustments to the flow of the office visit to achieve patient satisfaction. When Donna has time, she brings up the portal on her computer to research the side effects of the new medication, schedule an appointment with the neurologist and review her lab results.

Communication between doctor and patient that fosters information exchange and sets up proper expectations plays an important role in developing a trusting relationship, which correlates to the outcome of care. For centuries, hastily written notes taken during an office visit have made up a patient's health record and provided the basis for a treatment plan. Communication flow from doctor to patient began with a face-to-face meeting or a telephone conversation when the patient explained the problem and the doctor listened and then issued orders. There was little opportunity for discussion, questions, or debate. The fact that a doctor's decisions did not include much input from the patient seemed totally appropriate because most patients believed that their doctors were trained in medical school to make the right decisions for them.

In spite of the availability of the technology, not much seems to have changed. Well over two-thirds of doctors' offices use the same methods for recording and keeping patients records as they did 50 years ago, which is to say files full of paper and rooms filled with X-ray film. Most of those same doctors are still communicating with their patients via telephone and postal service.

Millions of doctor office visits occur every day across the world, and an intricate patchwork of information from providers and payers is processed for each visit. The records are on paper or housed in computer systems that typically have limited ability to exchange data electronically. And because those visits are only one aspect of healthcare that the individual experiences, the paperwork mounds in isolated files held by a myriad of medical professionals, including pharmacies, hospitals, labs, physical and occupational therapists, alternative medicine practitioners, dentists, specialists of all types, insurance companies, and private databases. These are typically files that did not communicate with one another.[1]

Scenario #1 depicts the traditional office visit that is infused with warmth and familiarity but lacking in communication between doctor and patient. Much of Eleanor's office visit time is spent watching the nurse and the doctor record information in her paper chart and ask questions about issues that she had already supplied on the update form. Facing lots of new problems – high blood pressure, high cholesterol – Eleanor has questions after her visit with no easy way to have them addressed. She resorts to an Internet search but is not quite sure about the reliability of the information she finds.

Scenario #2 depicts an office that has newly adopted communication technology to supply the doctor with quick answers and reference points. However, this office is not using these tools to foster better communication between the doctor and his patient. Dan still has the frustrating task of filling out an update form and trying to remember all of the important details of his medical history. During his visit, there are many awkward moments when the doctor is focused on the computer and not on Dan. Links to information resources are on paper and not the live links that patients are used to using.

Scenario #3 illustrates how use of communication technology (patient portal, email, PDA) can improve doctor/patient interaction during the office visit. Marie does not mind spending a few minutes before her visit updating her record on her patient portal. It is certainly better than filling in an update form. With the advance information sent to her PDA and the nurse's posts to the computer, Dr. Downes is able to give Donna her complete attention without the distraction of having to take notes. Email is the frosting on the cake that gives Donna a general sense of being well cared for, and gives Dr. Downes a sense of providing the best care available.

The twenty-first century healthcare consumer, who is an avid user of the Internet, email communication, and digital information, realizes that there is more to patient

---

[1] The Markle Foundation and the Robert Wood Johnson Foundation July 2004

care than engaging in a hurried conversation and receiving instructions from a qualified healthcare professional. With the availability of health information from print media, television, Internet resources, books, magazine articles, patients have high expectations that their healthcare experiences will include greater participation, two-way discussion and a means for follow up if they have questions. Patients want their experience with a physician to be warm, reassuring, and satisfying. They expect their doctors to be good listeners and to suggest appropriate information resources that help them learn more about treatments and options. Patients have a low tolerance for doctors who allow the telephone to interrupt them, who dismiss their ailments as incidental, and who avoid confronting difficult situations. They expect their physician to ask relevant questions and, through eye contact, body language, tempo of speech and tone of voice, to imply that this discussion has their full, undivided attention. That means no writing in paper charts and no typing on the computer.

Tommy Thompson U.S. Secretary of Health and Human Services from 2001–2005 stated during his tenure "grocery stores are more automated than the doctor's office." It is shockingly clear that the healthcare industry has lagged behind every other institution in deploying simple communication tools, email, cell telephones, personal digital assistants, text messaging and the Internet, that people use everyday in their home and work lives.

One of the ways that health information technology can be most effective is in generating reminders to patients about taking medication on time and all the time, and providing comprehensive, but understandable information about what a medication treats and how to properly administer it. Studies have proven that over 50% of individuals taking medication take their prescribed medications intermittently or discontinue them altogether. Forgetfulness, confusion about how to take a medication or why it is necessary, inability to pay for the prescription are all the reasons cited when patients are asked why they are not adhering to their doctor's instructions. Somewhere along the way, there is miscommunication when patients report that they are unclear about why they are taking a particular medication or why it is necessary to finish all the medication in the bottle once they are feeling better. Without a direct channel of communication to the doctor to clear up their confusion, most of the patients' failure to adhere compounds their problems. The telephone, with its frustrating tag is not an answer. Email with its fast response mechanism and the ability to provide live links that direct the patient to Websites that explain a medication and the reasons why it is important or offer comments by other patients suffering from the same condition can be an effective way to promote better adherence.

Over 40% of the American population has at least one chronic health condition (defined as a medical problem that lasts a year or longer, limits what a person can do, and requires ongoing care). Twenty percent have two or more such conditions and millions more are officially disabled. An individual practitioner or small group practice, using paper records, is not well equipped to care for these patients. They do not have the support staff, time, or tools to work with the patient and the family. Their medical record system is cumbersome and information is hard to access, making it difficult to track patients and provide them with the education they need.

The demands of a physician's daily practice make it difficult to reorganize and train staff in new communication tools such as electronic health records and patient portals, or to keep up with the latest discoveries, disease threats, and devices designed to help a physician offer twenty-first century quality medical care. There are no quick fixes. However, it is incumbent upon healthcare professionals to arm themselves and their patients with as much information as possible. This can be accomplished with current technology that enables access to vast information resources.

Digital Communication in Medical Practice is a guidebook that provides a quick comprehensive overview of the tools available to every practicing physician. The book illustrates how proven communication technology – the computer, email, PDAs, and the Internet can help doctors address the crunch of too little time, too many patients, and too much information. Authors, Nancy Finn, technologist and Bill Bria, doctor medical informatics expert, and communications expert spent two years talking with the early adopters, heads of medical institutions, private practitioners, insurers, employers, policymakers, and especially patients. The result is a book that focuses on how Electronic Health Records (EHR) and Personal Health Records (PHR) digitize patient information and make it easier for doctors and patients to collaboratively view and add data to the health record for continuity of care. This book discusses the convenience of using email and patient portals, to offer advice about post surgical care, nutrition, changing a medication, or discussing lab results. It points out how eliminating telephone tag and incorporating email and Web communications can result in less frequent office visits for those things that can be handled with a quick response, giving the doctor more time to see patients who truly have a need to be seen, and enabling the physician to have a more collaborative relationship with all patients.

Digital Communication in Medical Practice also discusses concerning issues of security, privacy, and healthcare quality, and outlines the legislative initiatives that have been passed to protect healthcare information from unauthorized entry. The book delves into perplexing, but critically important questions about the high cost of healthcare services and how various payment structures impact the doctor's ability to be paid a fair wage for professional services. The authors discuss how the Internet with its vast information resources quickly and efficiently enables physicians to find answers that result in better healthcare choices for patients. This book outlines how practitioners in remote locations can log onto the Internet, and, with simple tools such as telephones with cameras attached, can consult with super-specialists at major medical centers. It describes how homebound chronically ill patients can have their vital signs monitored 24/7 over the Internet. The inclusion of many anecdotal stories, using fictional names and settings, but based on real patient experiences, and case studies illustrates how these communication tools or the lack thereof can make a significant difference in treatment and outcome. A medical professional reading this book will come to understand that the introduction of digital communication into a practice including electronic health records, use of the Internet, e-prescribing, telemedicine, and other technologies will save time, money, and most importantly will reduce critical medical errors and thus save lives.

Chapter 1
eHealth and Patient Safety

*"Change involves the crystallization of new actions, possibilities
new policies, new behaviors, new patterns, new methodologies,
new products or new market ideas, based on reconceptualization
of old ones to make new and hopefully more productive actions
possible."*

Rosabeth Moss Kantor
The Change Masters, Simon and Schuster Touchstone
Division, 1984

*John, a Gulf War veteran with cancer, logs into his secure Web-based My HealtheVet
from home and receives updated laboratory results and information about a new
treatment. After reviewing the information John uses the My HealtheVet Web interface to access benefits and eligibility information and to schedule an appointment at
a community-based outpatient clinic close to his home.*

*Although he does not need them today, John also has access to electronic pre-
scription refills, cancer-specific health information and resources, and record for-
warding eServices for second opinions. He can review and upload clinical
information through a home monitoring unit and can authorize access to My
HealtheVet services for family members.*

*At a scheduled appointment with his physician, John shares treatment informa-
tion with his doctor and an oncologist from a renowned specialty cancer center
who participates in the discussion via videoconference. Based on a mutual decision
to pursue further treatment, John undergoes several tests to decide if he is an
appropriate candidate.*

*Once the test results are ready, John is alerted that they have been automatically
added to his electronic medical record and are available for viewing in his personal
health record (PHR). Using his Web interface, he reviews the results at home and
authorizes consent for the cancer center oncologist to make the results available to
a remote care team so treatment planning can begin.[1]*

Healthcare professionals have spent many years resisting change and holding onto
paper-based clinical record keeping, as well as insisting on face-to-face or telephone
communication with patients. Meanwhile, other industries throughout the world have
embraced computer technology and changed the way they interact with their clients

N.B. Finn and W.F. Bria, *Digital Communication in Medical Practice*,
DOI: 10.1007/978-1-84882-355-6_2, © Springer-Verlag London Limited 2009

and customers. In the transportation industry, there is no longer any paper. The eTicket is what you get. When you go to the car dealership to have your automobile serviced, all of the car's records are online so the technicians can see exactly what has been done and what is needed. Banks encourage their customers to access their bank statements online eliminating the mailed monthly copy. Travel itineraries are planned online; college courses are delivered via Web-based modules; entertainment tickets are ordered and delivered online. Even in the retail industry, the landscape is rapidly changing. When year-end shopping is tallied, more purchases are made online than traditional face-to-face store encounters.

EHealth programs with electronic storage, retrieval, management and communication of health information are finally taking hold. As an ePatient, John is proactive and works directly with his doctors to make decisions about his treatment plan. John's story illustrates that eHealth fosters a collaborative environment where there is sharing of information, interactive communication, patient empowerment, and improved patient safety. It is the patient safety issue that has forced health organizations to take a closer look at eHealth.

Medical Error: Woe is Me; Woe is You

Jerilyn, a patient at the Beth Israel Deaconess (BID) Medical Center in Boston, had been seeing an endocrinologist for a benign thyroid tumor. When she revisited the doctor for a check up, the clinical exam revealed that the tumor had shrunk or remained the same. Nevertheless, to be safe, the doctor recommended that Jerilyn get an ultrasound. Jerilyn had the ultrasound, and the next day utilized the BID patient site, where she was able to review her lab results. What she saw there shocked her. The radiology report indicated that the tumor had grown from a previous test. Since this was contrary to the clinical observation, Jerilyn pulled up her electronic record on her Patient Site. She realized that something did not compute. When she reviewed both tests she noted that either the radiologist had the wrong report or had the wrong patient, because the numbers from the earlier test did not match the numbers from the new test.

Jerilyn called her endocrinologist who was upset that she had seen her labs on Patient Site before he had a chance to review them. He told her to go into the hospital for a biopsy. Jerilyn called the radiologist who insisted that the report he had posted was correct. But she still had her doubts so Jerilyn put off the biopsy and went for an independent ultrasound that confirmed that there was a mistake in the posting and she did not need a biopsy. Her actions saved her from undergoing a procedure for no reason and saved the medical system multiple dollars.

Medical errors maim and kill more people per year than breast cancer, AIDS, or motor vehicle accidents."[2]

"The number of people who die annually in the United States from medical errors is higher than number of Americans who died in the Korean and Vietnam wars combined, as reported by official Pentagon sources."[3]

Although it is true that all human beings including medical professionals make mistakes, studies conducted by the Institute of Medicine have shown that as many as 40% of these mistakes are judged preventable![4]

Keeping Patients Safe

Nearly 50% of patients, when asked, say they are concerned about an error resulting in injury happening to themselves or to a member of their family when they receive care as an outpatient or when they go to a hospital for care.[5]

Patient safety problems of all types happen. Many are preventable. Some are inexcusable. All are unwarranted. Typically the errors do not result from individual recklessness but from flaws in health organizations. One of the most profound causes of medical error is lack of communication and information. Too often healthcare professionals are working with incomplete information about a patient at the point of care.

A study conducted by the Agency for Healthcare Policy and Research (AHCPR) found that missing clinical information might lead to adverse events and delays in services in outpatient primary care. AHRQ researchers collected point-of-care data during patient visits from 253 clinicians across 32 primary care practices on the type, frequency, and consequences of missing clinical information. Among 1,614 clinical visits, clinicians reported that important information was missing in 13.6% of cases (220 visits). Among these visits, the most common types of missing information were lab and radiology results (45% and 28.2%, respectively), letters or dictation containing clinical information (39.5%), and patient history or physical exam findings (26.8%). Clinicians reported that potential adverse outcomes due to missing clinical information were at least somewhat likely in 44% of these visits, and clinicians who use electronic medical records were significantly less likely to report missing clinical information than their peers with paper-based records. They found that computer systems detected 60 times as many adverse drug reactions in patients as the traditional method used at one hospital where the study was conducted. These computer-based systems also generate reminders for physicians related to monitoring and tracking patients, for example, administering flu vaccine or monitoring and adjusting medications.[6]

Missing clinical information can consume physicians' time and cause undue worry and grief for the physician and the patient (see Table 1.1). Gaps in information lead to prescribing medications that do not interact well with other prescriptions

Table 1.1 Common Preventable Medical Errors that Occur at the Point of Care

1.	Human error caused by illegible writing in medical records or on prescription orders.
2.	Failue to integrate clinical information systems.
3.	Inaccessibility of records.
4.	Lack of information about a patient's allergies.

the patient may be taking, potentially resulting in adverse reactions. Missing information can cause a misdiagnosis because the physician does not have all the facts at hand. It can lead to repeating tests, putting the patient through pain and stress and costing the system unnecessary, wasted dollars.

On February 22, 2000, Josie an 18-month-old baby girl was admitted to a prestigious East Coast hospital after suffering burns when she climbed into a hot bath. Her mother kept a day and night vigil at her bedside. While in the hospital, Josie became severely dehydrated and her mother heard the doctor tell the staff that Josie was not to receive any more pain medication. Shortly thereafter a nurse came in with a syringe filled with pain medication for Josie. The mother questioned the nurse who said the orders had been changed and she administered the injection. Fifteen minutes later Josie' heart stopped and she suffered cardiac arrest. Two days later Josie was taken off life support and died in her mother's arms. Her death was preventable.

Here is obvious case of miscommunication and misunderstanding that led to the death of a child. In response to this horrific event, Josie's family set up the Josie King Foundation. The Foundation has three programs to promote patient safety:

1. **Condition H** to address the needs of the patient and family in case of an emergency or when the patient is unable to get the attention of a healthcare provider in an emergency situation. A patient or a member of the patient's family calls a Condition H signaling the need for immediate help when they feel they are not receiving adequate medical attention or are concerned. Within minutes of a Condition H call a rapid response team arrives at the patient's bedside Members of the team include internal medicine house physician, a patient relations coordinator, and a nursing coordinator and floor staff. The program has been pioneered at the University of Pittsburgh Medical Center and affiliated hospitals.
2. **Care Journal**, a tool to help patients and their family record the details of their medical care and help them better manage their care while in the hospital. The Care Journal has prompts to help the patient use it effectively. Any individual who might need to go into the hospital can request a Care Journal free of charge at the Josie King website http://www.josieking.org.
3. The Foundation has also established the **Josie King Nursing Awards Fund** to support nursing studies that focus on improving patient safety and reducing harm. This Fund is administered by the Johns Hopkins Department of Nursing.

A 71-year-old woman with congestive heart failure was admitted to the hospital. She did not have a preadmission diagnosis of diabetes. In the emergency room, she had a routine blood test and her blood sugar was elevated. At 11:30 pm, the nurse notified the covering intern who ordered an insulin dosage to be given to her. At 1:10 am, her blood sugar was checked once again by a different nurse and was elevated even more. The intern ordered more insulin. At 3:00 am, another blood test was taken and the intern ordered more insulin. At 11:00 am, the next morning a different covering intern was notified that this woman's blood sugar level continued to rise and 8 units of insulin were given intravenously. At 3:40 pm, the patient was unresponsive and another blood check revealed low blood sugar. Later it was discovered that many of the blood specimens had been drawn incorrectly, resulting in a higher reading than the actual condition of the patient. Fortunately, the patient suffered no lasting harm.[7]

This case highlights the challenges of cross coverage and the management of this patient by three healthcare workers who were not familiar with her. It points out the difficulties experienced by medical workers who do not have a complete history of the patient and a full assessment of the patient's problems. Twenty-first century digital communication tools, especially an eHealth record that follows the patient wherever treated, are now available to address such communication gaps and provide a safer healthcare environment.

The eHealth Triangle

The eHealth Professional

Health begins with the eHealth professional - a twenty-first century practicing medical professional who is plugged in and online. EHealth professionals use electronic health records, online databases, e-Prescribing, email and portals, to reduce

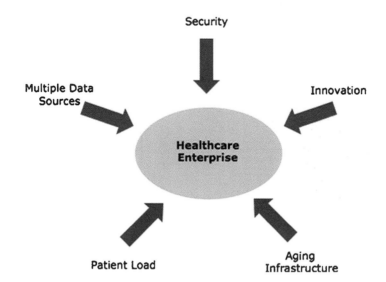

Figure 1.1 Challenges driving eHealth applications
Depicts the complexity of the healthcare system and the many factors that impact eHealth as the way to deliver care.

medical error, and increase patient safety. With electronic health records, eHealth professionals should not experience gaps in information at the point of care. A proper EHR is constantly updated and goes with the patient wherever and whenever that patient requires care. With digital databases and a PDA, eHealth professionals have the diagnostic triggers and decision support tools to cull out the proper diagnosis at the patient's beside, in the clinic or in the office. With a simple camera attached to a digital telephone communication system, eHealth professionals in an urban or remote area can work with colleagues at major medical centers to address complex conditions and unexpected emergencies. With patient portals and email, eHealth professionals can stay in touch with patients, especially those who suffer from chronic conditions and require the type of daily monitoring that can be done via computer and communications tools directly to a healthcare professional. These ongoing communications enable patients and eHealth professionals to make adjustments in medications and talk through issues, keeping these patients out of the emergency room.

Online communication between physicians and patients has been increasing (see Figure 1.2) since 2004, with nearly 30 million consumers reporting that they connect online with a physician today. Thirty-one percent of all physicians report that they communicate online with patients; the majority of such physicians perform clinical activities with patients online. Online communications includes email, instant messaging, or secure messaging services.

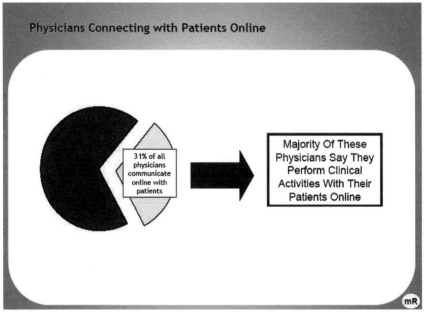

© Manhattan Research

Figure 1.2   Physicians connecting with patients online

The eHospital

There are many hospitals that have implemented digital communication technology tools to admit, track, and treat patients. These eHospitals strategically place computers throughout their physical plant so that their eHealth Professionals can enter information, access information, and track patients in a variety of locations including: the admissions offices, the ER, the ICU, and the patient floor. The eHospital's information systems and bar code technology enables eHealth Professionals to manage and reduce the number of medication errors with scanning of the medication container and the patient's wristband.

The Brigham and Women's Hospital in Boston MA, using barcode technology realized an 85% drop in medication errors when prescriptions orders were moved from paper to a bar code system.[8]

In the eHospital, information systems provide clinicians with widespread access to digital radiology images whether they are at their office, in the hospital, or in a remote location, enabling them to make accurate diagnoses quickly and efficiently. EHospitals also have an advantage when faced with disaster recovery. Unlike the weeks and in some cases months that it took healthcare professionals in New Orleans to restore patient records following the Katrina floods in 2005, eHospitals, with appropriate off site back up systems, can restore electronic patient records in a matter of hours, if they were to lose their primary data center.

Case Study: The VA has HIT Covered

The $18.3 billion Veterans Administration is the nation's largest integrated hospital and healthcare system. It includes over 172 hospitals, 600 outpatient clinics, 132 nursing homes, 206 counseling centers, 73 home healthcare agencies and assorted other programs. As Hurricane Katrina flooded the streets of New Orleans, VA hospital employees, located near the Superdome - did not have to worry about lugging thousands of patient folders to higher ground, because they knew their electronic patient record's system was secure. The Veterans Health Information Systems and Technology Architecture program, or VistA, captures patient information and makes it available for clinical and administrative tasks at any VA medical facility. As the veterans who were patients in New Orleans were airlifted to VA hospitals in Houston and other locations in the South, the center's VistA backup tapes were transported along with them.

The VA system stands out as having one of the most automated eHospitals in the world. When the doctors at the VA hospitals make rounds, they do so with a laptop computer on a portable cart where they enter notes right at the patient's bedside. VA doctors use PDAs that have a database of the patient's barcoded information, and they match that to the patient identification barcode on the wristband. All medications also have their own bar code identification. Before medicating a patient, a nurse or staff member laser scans three barcodes: the one in the computer, the one on the medication, and the one on the patient's wrist. The scans are entered into the computer. In a few seconds, software verifies that the right person is receiving the right drug in the right dose at the right time. The program screens for other potential problems such as drug interactions. If everything checks out, the software simply records the event in the patient's electronic record. If not, it flashes an immediate warning. The system makes it very hard to give the patient the wrong medication. With this program, the VA has experienced a sixfold reduction in medication errors.

A key digital communication feature at the VA is the reminder system - pop ups that prompt the physician to perform certain labs or measurements. In monitoring a patient with potential hypertension, for example, the system reminds the doctor that a blood pressure reading is due. If a patient has a preexisting condition such as diabetes, it reminds the doctor to get a Hemoglobin A1 test done and it can be ordered with just one click.[9]

Hospital chief information officers have had a long history of fighting to convince healthcare CFOs that information technology initiatives are mission critical to patient safety. The VA case illustrates how much impact health information technology can have. In the hospital environment where there is often a need for split second information exchange among doctors, nurses, and staff, the availability of the right information at the right time can mean the difference between comfort and suffering, even life and death for the patient. Shortages of nurses and other staff, a universal problem in healthcare, has made it increasingly clear that medical teams must work within a framework that synchronizes communications and records-keeping into a fully transparent system, one that provides the physician with up to date patient information and analysis, whether that patient is in the doctor's office in the hospital, visiting a lab or an outpatient hospital-based clinic.

Case Study: The Dana Farber Cancer Institute

The death of two cancer patients at the Dana Farber Cancer Institute, in Boston, who were both administered poisonous doses of a chemotherapy medication, in 1995 caused a public outcry that forced significant changes and adoption of technology at that institution. One of the women, a reporter for the Boston Globe, died immediately as a result of the error. The other woman suffered permanent heart damage and died several months later. Since those fatal events, corrective eHealth actions were taken that include:

1. Doctors are not allowed to hand write prescriptions any longer since the mistaken doses were from handwritten orders.
2. Once the information from the doctor goes into the computer, it is matched with the upper dose limits for the drug and other preprogrammed guidelines. If the doctor makes a mistake the system signals the error.

3. A nurse checks the information in the computer before ordering a drug from the pharmacy.
4. The pharmacist conducts another computerized review checking for drug interactions and patient allergies.
5. Once the drug is prepared and sent to the patient floor, the drug goes to the nurses' station where two nurses check the drug's label and the patient's wristband barcode to make sure the right person is getting the right drug.[10]

Reducing Errors in the Emergency Department

In all emergency departments, the potential for medical error is enormous. The fast response and critical care nature of the ER means, the staff is working under extremely stressful conditions. This environment is quite similar to the aviation industry, where the air traffic controllers and pilots work in a high stress and fast-paced industry that requires exacting standards. In response to a series of accidents and errors, the aviation industry developed data analysis programs for collecting and analyzing safety-related data and adopted a reporting approach that is nonpunitive, confidential, and independent of any authority or oversight group. They also developed training tools - The Crew Resource Management (CRM) training program to improve safety for flight crews. CRM focuses on teaching crew members to recognize and understand cognitive errors and shows them how stressors such as fatigue, emergencies, and work overload contribute to the occurrence of errors. CRM, which has reduced the number of plane crashes, has been adopted by many healthcare organizations and is showing great promise in reducing postsurgical mortality rates.[11]

Case Study: The Dashboard at BIDMC

Recognizing the need to address the overflow of patients and the shortages of staff faced by every large urban hospital, the Beth Israel Deaconess Medical Center in Boston, MA (BIDMC), created a special workflow system, the Dashboard, similar to that used by airport traffic controllers. This system uses computer monitors to tell the healthcare professionals which patients are coming in, who is languishing in a delay pattern, and where all patients are located. It includes patient admitting information, a full discharge summary, all medication information, and other relevant medical history that has traditionally been on a paper chart. A wireless cell phone network enables the attending physicians, interns, or residents to communicate to physicians outside the hospital and keeps everyone informed about each patient. If a patient arrives unconscious but has a driver's license, the staff can access pharmacy information and patient treatment records by tracking the license through to the patient's medical insurance provider. Built into the Dashboard is an EKG machine locator that enables the ER staff to identify where their equipment is being used and triage it to the most vital cases. Every BIDMC ER doctor carries a cell phone that is part of the internal network so the doctors can communicate with one another immediately. On the cell phone system, there is a special number that rings to a senior physician if there is a need for a consult. All prescriptions at BIDMC are electronically stored so if the emergency room visitor is a patient of the hospital, medication records are immediately accessible.[12]

ePatients

Asking patients to adopt technology tools is not the problem in the eHealth world. Most patients are online and avid users of email that is a constant in their lives. They surf the Internet daily for many types of information including health information. The Pew Internet & American Life Project reports that 52 million American adults rely on the Internet to make critical health decisions; 73 million American adults use the Internet to research prescription drugs and explore new ways to control their weight and search for other health information. On any given day, approximately 6 million Americans go online for medical advice that means that more people go online for healthcare-related issues than actually visit health professionals. These ePatients typically look for answers to specific questions. They use this information to enlighten themselves in preparation for a visit to their physicians. The PEW research report indicates that 61% of ePatients who use the Internet report that the Internet has improved the way they take care of their own health, or take care of their loved ones.[13]

For millions of patients who suffer from chronic diseases, PEW research found over 75% of the individuals that they surveyed reported that information that they find in an Internet search affected a decision about how to treat their illness or condition. For some individuals, the information led them to ask their physician new questions or get a second opinion; others reported that the information they found changed the way they cope with a chronic condition or manage their pain. Over 50% indicated that the information they found in an Internet search changed their overall approach to their health or the health of someone they take care of.[14]

In spite of their personal use of eTools, ePatients continue to tolerate doctors who rely on paper for keeping their records, telephone calls for answering their questions, and snail mail for communicating test results. However, many ePatients are generating their own personal health records and are actively requesting that their doctors get into the wired world and consider electronic health records. Many are also insisting that their eHealth professionals communicate with them via email. Today's ePatients want to partner with their healthcare professionals in determining together the best possible approach for a specific problem. They want their PCP to coordinate their care with specialists and alternative healthcare providers. As they move from institution to institution, ePatients want their information to move with them seamlessly. All of this is dependent upon digital communication.

eHealth Around the World

Worldwide, the eHealth landscape is changing. A shift in attention, interest and resources toward the implementation of Internet-related healthcare activities and the use of emerging information and communication to improve or enable better, safer patient care is no longer an anomaly and many countries have adopted health information technology, albeit in different and varied formats.

Europe

In Sweden community, nursing assistants carry PDAs with mobile drug management software links in real time to Sweden's national Fass.se online drug database. This helps these nurses identify adverse drug reactions among their elderly patients. The nursing assistants' PDAs are also equipped with bar code scanners. When they arrive at the home of a patient, they are able to scan all of the medicine packages to get a correct picture of what the patient is taking. They can check these medications in the Fass database. This audit enables them to check on whether the drugs are suitable and whether there are contraindications among the drugs prescribed and used.[15]

In Germany, nearly 2,000 patients with chronic heart problems and 200 with diabetes are monitored at home by wearing devices that look at their blood pressure or blood sugar levels and trigger a warning that is sent through the telephone to healthcare personnel at the Public Health Telemedicine Service located in Düsseldorf. These patients are monitored 24/7 and if their readings are not satisfactory, the patient receives a call within 5 min. If the reading is classified as an emergency, the patient's physician is contacted and an ambulance is sent. This telemedicine application has reduced hospital admissions by 50% as well as dramatically improving the life and security of these patients.[16]

In Italy, a National Electronic Health Programme launched in 2004 is slowly bringing electronic health records, telemedicine, and a national online booking system to the healthcare industry.[17]

In the United Kingdom, healthcare is delivered to citizens through the National Health Service. Early on NHS initiated the NHSDO (Direct Online Division) service to provide citizens and healthcare professionals with access to information about healthcare via the Internet. The NHSDO is a Web portal offering citizens information to help them understand health, healthcare issues, and services including advice on nutrition, self-treatment guides, and healthcare services available by region, best treatments Websites, FAQs, and interactive tools. The idea is to empower citizens of the UK and encourage them to be full partners in their healthcare.[18]

Another UK program fosters patient use of smart mobile phones to create and access a personal health record as well as to have a video consultation with their physician.[19]

The Amsterdam Health Service has developed a Web-based patient clinic that offers easy anonymous screening for people at risk of sexually transmitted diseases (STDs). Visitors to the Website register with a pseudonym and are then able to print a referral letter, which entitles them to an anonymous free of charge blood sample to be taken at one of seven laboratories in Amsterdam. Following this, the laboratory posts the results online where they can be accessed by the individual. Should the test prove positive, the patient is advised to visit an STD clinic for diagnosis, confirmation, and treatment.[20]

In the Czech Republic, citizens enjoy an electronic health record in which they are full participants combined with Internet access in a system called IZIP. The EHR includes relevant information about patient visits with a GP, dental treatments, laboratory, and imaging services. With the consent of the patient, the IZIP system allows doctors to access the patient EHR at the point of care. Patients have the right to access and add to their EHR but cannot change the record. They can authorize healthcare professionals to view and update their data. The system helps patients and healthcare professionals work together to make responsible decisions about their treatment.[21]

Asia

Investments in healthcare-related information systems have been on the rise across Asia-Pacific as both government and private healthcare organizations rollout plans for achieving "electronic hospital status."

In India, a large telemedicine initiative connecting several very small towns and villages with major specialty hospitals provides people with care they could not otherwise receive during a crucial emergency or accident. This project links leading hospitals in India, via mobile V-Sats. General practitioners in those local towns and villages participate in live interactive consultations with specialists at a prefixed time. The system includes Store and Forward consultations, where the local general practitioner forwards patient records and diagnostic test reports, and receives the specialist's opinion enabling him to gives the diagnoses to the patient at a later time. The idea is to move clinical information rather than the patient."[22]

The Hong Kong Hospital Authority (HKHA) is one of a handful of organizations world-wide that have made great progress with an IT-based clinical management system and a single, comprehensive electronic patient records system for its seven million patients. These systems are used daily by all 30,000 clinical workers in all its facilities. National Healthcare Group doctors no longer write out prescriptions manually. All prescriptions are electronically entered and transmitted to the pharmacies eliminating paper and errors at the same time.

One major achievement is the development of their clinical management system (CMS). CMS is used daily by all the 30,000 staff under HKHA. In addition to recording patients' medical history, the CMS also improves patient protection. The additional clinical decision support function provides nurses and clinicians the drug-to-food and drug-to-drug interaction alerts.

Leveraging the success of CMS, HKHA has extended the access of these medical records to the private sector. The electronic patient record system (EPR) caught a lot of media attention regarding patients' privacy when it was first introduced. To enhance the system's security and patients' privacy, medical records of patients, who have agreed to participate in the EPR, are transferred to a secured data warehouse. The records are only available for private doctors through a "three-factor authentication" process.[23]

The IT team of Singapore Health Services (SingHealth, which oversees public-sector healthcare institutions in the eastern zone of Singapore) has built a network of digital hospitals, national specialist centers and polyclinics. The implementation of the outpatient administrative system (OAS), which involved 16 clinical organizations in the SingHealth system, was completed in 2006. They have also integrated nine polyclinics' databases into one. This initiative provides better clinical care by improving communication between specialist centers and hospitals and enabling the sharing of patient demographics, medical alerts, allergies, and billing information. X-ray images are also captured, stored, and accessed digitally.[24]

Key Points

1. The significant negative impact of medical error has been a driver for the implementation of digital communication in healthcare. The goal is to avoid unnecessary problems, and insure that healthcare professionals have all the information they need at the point of care.
2. EHealth that includes electronic storage, retrieval management, and communication of information provides a collaborative healthcare environment where information is shared by patients and providers.
3. The three prongs of eHealth: the eHealth professional, the eHospital, and the ePatient depend upon the existence of electronic health records and digital databases for safer, more efficient, less costly healthcare across a variety of populations.
4. EHealth is changing the healthcare landscape worldwide with great promise and variety in approach.

References and Notes

1. Story adapted from a HealtheVet use case scenario, written by Douglas Goldstein and reprinted permission from the VA and from the Markle Foundation.
2. Centers for Disease Control and Prevention National Center for Health Statistics Deaths: Preliminary Data for 1998, 1999. National vital Statistics Reports, Washington DC Department of Health and Human Services.
3. Rosemary Gibson and Janardan Presad Singh. Wall of Silence The Untold Story of the Medical Mistakes That Kill and Injure Millions of Americans. Lifeline Press; 2003:41.
4. To Err is Human: Building A Safer Health System. Washington: National Academy Press; 2000:33.
5. Kaiser Family Foundation Health Poll, July/August 2003.
6. Project Title: Applied Strategies for Improving Patient Safety Research Area: R-DEMO AHRQ Grant: HS11878 Principal Investigator: Wilson Pace, MD Reference: Smith   PC, Araya-Guerra R, Bublitz C, Parnes B, Van Vorst R, Westfall JM, Pace WD. Missing clinical information during primary care visits. *JAMA*, 2005;2935:565–571
7. http:22webmm.ahrq.gov/case.aspx
8. Brigham to Adopt Barcodes to Cut Errors by Liz Kowalczyk, The Boston Globe March 16, 2006, www.boston.com/business/articles/2005/03/16/
9. Interview with Ross Fletcher Chief of Staff VA Medical Center, Washington, DC. "A Government Health System Leads the Way" by Lani Luciano Reducing Medical Errors and Improving Patient Safety: Success Stories form the Front Lines of Medicine, The National Coalition on Health Care: The Institute for Healthcare Improvement, February 2000.
10. AHRQ webM&M: Case and Commentary, http://webmmm.ahrq.gov/perspective. aspx?perspectiveID=3
11. Ruchlin HS, Dubbs NL, Callahan MA. The role of leadership in instituting a culture of safety: Lessons from the literature. *Journal of Healthcare Management* 2004;49(1):47.
12. Based on tour and interview with Larry Nathanson M.D. Director of Emergency Medicine Informatics, the Beth Israel Deaconess.
13. PEW Internet & American Life Vital Decisions: How Internet Users Decide What Information to Trust when they or their Loved Ones are Sick, Susannah Fox, Director of Research May 2002:4-6. www.perinternet.org
14. "EPatients with a Disability or Chronic Disease", Susannah Fox, PEW Internet & American Life Project p.ii
15. "PDA Software Lets Nursing Assistants Review Drugs," October 24, 2007 eHealth Europe Media Ltd. http://ehealtheurope.net/news/3150/.
16. eHealth Europe "Telemedicine Growing in Use in Germany" eHealth Media Ltd, June 2007 http://ehealtheurope.net/new/2787/telemedicine
17. eHealth Europe "Italy's National Electronic Health Programme" eHealth Media Ltd, June 2007 http://ehealtheurope.net/features/item.cfm?docld = 201
18. eHealth Impact 7.9 DG INFSO October 2006 www.nhsdirect.uk, www.eHealth-impact.org/ case_studies/index_en.htm
19. eHealth Europe "3G Doctor Launches Videophone Consultations" eHealth Media Ltd, October 2007, www.e-health-insider.com/news/3132
20. www.ehealtheurope.net/news/3114 E-Health Europe: "Amsterdam to Launch STD Clinic Online Oct. 2007.
21. eHealth Impact 7.5 DG INFSO October 2006 www.pzip.czwww.ehealth-impact.org/case_studies/index_en.htm
22. The Economic Times "Moire V-sat Mobile Units to Connect Hospital Network Oct 11, 2007 http://economictimes.indiatimes.com
23. Healing hands by Susan Tsang published: Saturday, 1 September 2007 MIS Magazine, Asia www.misweb.com Source: Hong Kong Hospital Authority Senior IT executive: Andre Greyling, CIO
24. Singapore Health Services Senior IT executive: Fong Choon Khin, group chief technology officer Screens: 8,523 website: www.singhealth.com.sg

Chapter 2
New Health Care Models

"By computerizing health records, we can avoid dangerous
medical mistakes, reduce costs and improve care."

President George Bush, State of the Union Address, Jan. 20, 2004

Dr. Jacobs, who practices medicine in Davidson TN, is scheduled to see Anita, a
55-year-old accountant who works at the local university. During his busy office
hours, Dr. Jacobs sees a patient every 20 min. Today, however, Dr. Jacobs has an
issue that he has not faced before. He cannot locate Anita's chart.

When Anita walks into the office, she is asked, as usual, to fill out an update
form. Normally Dr. Jacobs glances quickly at the form to see if there is anything
new. Today, however, he has to take 10 min out of his busy schedule to review the
form thoroughly so that he has baseline information for this visit. Anita is a com-
plicated patient with issues that include rheumatoid arthritis and lung disease
caused by heavy smoking. With the update form in hand, Dr. Jacobs has a list of the
medications Anita is taking, and allergies that she included. However, he has no
idea about her most recent tests, inoculations, referrals to specialists, the calls she
has made to the nurse practitioner between visits and the results of her most recent
labs. In the 20 minutes allotted to the visit Dr. Jacobs has to spend much of the time
asking Anita basic questions about information that should be in the record. As a
result, he barely has time to discuss Anita's immediate concerns. Anita leaves the
office surprised that Dr. Jacobs remembers so little about her and her health. She
is also frustrated that there is not enough time for her to talk in more depth about
what is on her mind, which she considers to be legitimate concerns.

This anecdote reflects why the practice of twenty-first century medicine calls for
twenty-first century information management in the form of an electronic health
record that is available 24/7 wherever the doctor is seeing a patient – in his office,
at a nursing home in the hospital, or at the patient's home. This record is kept in a
computer system and can be accessed at a terminal, with a laptop computer, desktop
computer or personal digital assistant (PDA). In an ideal situation, the electronic
health record's contents are backed up daily at an off-site location to prevent the
loss of patient information.

N.B. Finn and W.F. Bria, *Digital Communication in Medical Practice,*
DOI: 10.1007/978-1-84882-355-6_3, © Springer-Verlag London Limited 2009

There is evidence that in over 25% of patient visits to the doctor, where a paper chart constitutes the patient's health record, these charts are not available during the time of the patient appointment. Further when the doctor makes notes on a pad of paper during the office visit, that information has to be entered into the chart at a later time by the doctor or an office assistant. Often it doest not get there at all. Aside from the possibility that a paper chart can be misplaced, the sheer amount of medical information about each patient has increased so much over the past few years that it is difficult to manage unless it is in a digital format. There can be as many as 20 tests – blood work, X-rays, EKG, urinalysis, etc., associated with a single office visit, each with information that the doctor has to manage, record and communicate to the patient. It is not only the volume of information that is overwhelming. Patients expect that the doctor will have instant access to their record, just as they have instant access to information in their jobs or on their home computers.

Neither doctors nor patients in the twenty-first century would tolerate a bank that uses a paper-based process for depositing money, where the bank teller writes down the data for the deposit in a notebook and then transfers that information to several accounting books by hand. When the customer comes to the bank to make a withdrawal, the teller would have to search through all those paper documents to find out whether or not there is enough money in the account to enable the customer to take out the desired sum. Obviously, this system would be full of human errors and create intolerable frustration and delays. Fortunately, the banking industry automated those functions a long time ago, as have many service industries. Most auto service dealers, for example, can access an automobile's service history faster than a doctor, who is still working with a paper chart, can access a patient's health and treatment history. The paper-based healthcare system is fraught with errors and delays. It is time for change.

Continuous Available Information on Every Patient

The new eHealth medical infrastructure that includes electronic health records (EHRs), set up and maintained by clinicians, computer physician order entry (CPOE) where doctors enter orders directly into a computer, rather than issuing hand written orders, and personal health records (PHRs) that patients create to maintain information about their medical conditions: observations, actions taken, referrals to specialists, solutions such as medications, exercise and nutrition programs, obviates many of the problems described in these stories. Healthcare is complex and the prodigious amount of health information in the twenty-first century healthcare system makes digitization essential.

The Electronic Health Record is a digital software package that includes patient demographics, progress notes, problems, and medications, vital signs, past medical history, immunizations, laboratory data, radiology reports, and images. Many EHRs also include electronic provider notes, electronic viewing of laboratory and radiology results and electronic prescribing. The ability to exchange information across organizations known as health information exchange (HIE) or to collect electronic data for disease analysis are other components of many EHRs. Some EHR systems enable integration of complementary applications such as e-prescribing, referral management, and evidence-based decision support. One of the great benefits of an EHR is its ability to search all information in a patient's record and, based on best medical practice, (decision support tools) provide the physician with alerts ranging from fairly simple notices regarding immunizations or recommended screening tests, to more complex issues. For example, by analyzing a patient's history (or family history), most EHRs can identify the need for additional tests, prior to making a diagnosis or treatment recommendation.[1]

With an Electronic Health Record, the patient's office visit is a vastly different experience than it is used to be. With a few keystrokes, the healthcare professional can view comments from prior visits, lab tests, treatments, medications, notes from consults with specialists. If the patient has visited the emergency department between office visits, or was hospitalized, the EHR system, assuming that it interoperates with the health records at the hospital where the clinician has admitting rights, will have all of the notes, medications, tests, and diagnoses related to those occurrences.

Nearly eight out of 10 adults responding to a survey (see Figure 2.1) conducted by Deloitte said they are interested in having online access to their medical records and test results, and 26% said they would be willing to pay extra for the service, according to a September 2007 survey of 3,031 adults by Deloitte. Just 6% of respondents said they have accessed their medical records and test results online.

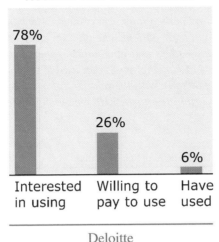

Deloitte

Figure 2.1 Are consumers interested in having online access to their medical records and test results? (C) 2008 Deloitte Development LLC. All rights reserved

EHR in the Hospital Setting

A survey conducted by the American Hospital Association (AHA) in 2006 revealed that an increasing number of hospitals are embracing health information technology and EHRs to improve quality, safety, and efficiency. Sixty-nine percent of responding hospitals reported they have either fully or partially implemented EHRs. Larger, urban, and teaching hospitals were more likely to have fully implemented EHR systems, and accounted for 11% of the total that responded to this survey.

Among the benefits of EHR are that they encourage physicians to order tests, labs, and medications electronically. Furthermore, EHR systems vastly improve charge capture and billing submissions to insurers that can be completed digitally within hours of treatment rather than days. All too frequently using manual systems, physicians' care in some hospitals never gets submitted for reimbursement. The EHR also helps hospital workers track treatment and provide the appropriate coding for accurate billing. The lack of interoperability between EHRs and other IT systems in the hospital poses the greatest challenge.

Driving the Adoption of the EHR in Small Group and Solo Practices

There are several factors that make EHR adoption desirable as shown in Table 2.1.

A group of vascular surgeons in Kentucky used to end their long day with two hours of paperwork, trying to read scribbled notes, dictating letters and document- ing the previous eight hours of patient visits. Months later when the patients returned to the office, the physicians would have a difficult time accessing that information. Then the office installed an electronic medical record system. Now each morning the doctors in the group access their EMR home page and view their inbox (patient notes) and their patient schedule. By electronically managing their schedule, messages and orders and eliminating paper documents and the ineffi- ciencies of manual record-keeping, the group is able to more accurately and effi- ciently care for their patients. With the addition of a scanner, staff assistants are able to digitize and incorporate into the EHR electronic versions of paper documents

Table 2.1 Factors that Make EHR Adoption Desirable

1.	Tickler file reminders for better care of patients with chronic health issues.
2.	Decision support and clinical practice guidelines built in.
3.	Faster transmission of patient information to and from laboratories, pharmacies, other specialists.
4.	Reporting functions that enable group practices to analyze trends related to chronic disease or notify patients of a medicine recall quickly and easily.
5.	Faster more efficient transcription of notes taken during the patient visit.
6.	Reduction in the number of unneeded office visits.
7.	Better, faster communication with patients–reduction of telephone tag.
8.	Direct links to information databases to help patients understand their medical issues.

*that other specialists and healthcare professionals send to the group on a patient's
behavior. They also now keep surgical images in this same electronic file.²*

Eliminating the burden of translating the notes from a patient visit, enjoying the
efficiency of having patient information available at all times, having a tickler file
for follow up procedures, and getting rid of the piles of paper and images on their
desk are reasons why this group of physicians and many others who have installed
EHRs have become advocates for this technology. When a physician writes a note
in the paper chart with a reminder to be sure the patient has a follow up chest X-ray
before the next office visit, that note is buried in the chart and is often forgotten.
That same note plugged into the EHR ties to a software-generated tickler that will
automatically remind the physician to notify the patient about having the chest
X-ray before the next visit. When the patient comes to see the doctor, the digital X-ray
is in the computer in front of the physician and together the doctor and the patient
can review the film and determine the next course of action. EHRs also provide
physicians or physician assistants with the ability to capture and transmit patient
information seamlessly to other specialists, labs, and pharmacies. They offer the
physician access to decision support and clinical practice guidelines – a robust database
of best practices for various conditions and illnesses. The physician can access these
clinical practice guidelines when making a decision on how to treat a patient who
presents with a number of symptoms that may not be straightforward. This capability
in the electronic health record offers the physician appropriate options to make good
choices based on best practices. In group practices, EHRs allow a practice to run reports
on thousands of patients without having to pull charts, enabling practice associates,
for example, to quickly notify people taking certain drugs if there has been a recall.
They can also track how many people in the practice may have a specific chronic
disease for which there are new discoveries that could benefit their patients.³

Case Study: Group Health Cooperative

*Group Health Cooperative (GHC), a private health care organization that insures
and provides care to 550,000 patients in Washington State, implemented their EHR
in 2003 and functions today in a completely " paperless" environment. All of doctors
at GHC engage in secure messaging with patients and 20% of patient visits with
primary care physicians are virtual. Matthew Handley, Internist and the Medical
Director of Informatics at Group Health Cooperative in Seattle, Washington, reports
that having digital health records mean fewer unnecessary office visits. Patients who
contact him often are seeking information and direction, not necessarily asking to be
seen. With the EHRs, Dr. Handley reports that he is able to identify and resolve problems more quickly and efficiently and those patients who opt to be seen can be scheduled in the same day, not days or weeks later. If the doctor is at home, in his office or
at any of the emergency rooms attached to hospitals in the area, the patient record is
instantly available to any doctor in the network. If a GHC patient travels out of state
and has an emergency, the doctor at a distant hospital can phone the on-call doctors
at GHC who access that patient's complete history and offer immediate assistance.
Although patients cannot change or alter their medical record, GHC doctors educate*

their patients to add data to their EHR whenever they have a new healthcare issue. Patients are also asked to review and update their record once a year. The EHR software automatically sends a written notation to the doctor that the patient has entered data into the record. Any condition that needs to be followed is flagged, so it will be noticed by a member of the patient's healthcare team. The GHC system provides a link to the Healthwise database where patients can research and find vast data and information on a healthcare issue that concerns them, empowering the patient and enabling patients and doctors to work together on a problem.[4]

Kathy Smith DiJulio, who has been a GHC patient for over 30 years and was a nurse there for 10 years, has experienced the full transition from a paper-based environment to the fully automated systems that she now enjoys as a patient. Her observations reinforce the benefits of The GHC approach to integrating digital communication technology in a medical practice. "It is wonderful to be away from telephone tag and to be able to get lab reports immediately. The system also provides me with full online access to the Healthwise knowledge database that I use to learn more about conditions that I have. In one situation I was going to ignore a symptom, but my research on the Healthwise database convinced me to seek immediate treatment that saved me much distress."

Installation, Implementation, and Impediments

Although there are many benefits to having an electronic health record, there are as many issues and reasons why this digital technology has been so slow to take hold (see Figure 2.2). The major barriers to universal adoption of EHRs are financial and

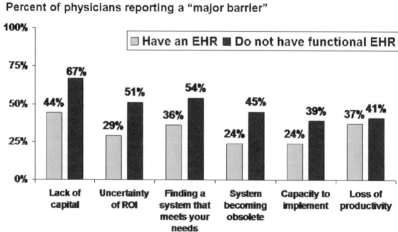

DesRoches CM, Campbell, EC, Rao SR, Donelan K, Ferris TG, Jha A, Kaushal R, Levy D, Rosenbaum S, Shields A, Blumenthal D. Electronic Health Records in Ambulatory Care – A National Survey of Physicians. New England Journal of Medicine©.

Figure 2.2 Major barriers to EHR implementation

cultural. Implementing an electronic health record is an expensive venture, particularly for the small practice with five or fewer full-time physicians. The costs of EHRs vary from $1,000 per physician in a group practice to up to $50,000 per physician. This is a huge variation and is chiefly based on how much customization of the software is required, the hardware expenditure required, and the configuration that the practice chooses (see Table 2.2).

There are three ways to acquire EHRs and the choice is dependent upon the cost, time, staff involved in the implementation and the need for interconnection between a single group practice and others with whom the group interacts such as hospitals, specialists in the area, labs, pharmacies, etc.

1. The Stand-alone model is an EHR that is used by a solo or very small group practice. It does not communicate or exchange information with other systems and essentially automates the record-keeping function within that office. It can be a robust EHR with all of the bells and whistles including decision support tools but it operates only to digitize information for that practice and does not have health information exchange capabilities.
2. The Application Service Provider (**ASP**) model is a subscription service model where the practice contracts for services from an outside vendor who provides the EHR and takes care of all of the related needs for an EHR implementation including support, maintenance, and training. The practice typically pays a monthly fee to the ASP provider. The chief advantages of the ASP model are lower capital outlay and start up costs, strong support, and a much more rapid implementation. With the ASP model, the time and frustration inherent in an implementation of

Table 2.2 Factors to Consider in Adopting an EHR for a Group or Solo Practice

1.	Willingness of the entire group of doctors to adapt to and use the system, i.e. getting buy-in from everyone.
2.	Hardware compatibility with the software purchase of an EHR.
3.	Knowing where the money for the system will come from.
4.	Understanding what it takes to train physicians and staff including: the cost of training consultants, time away from the practice, requirements for updates and retraining of new staff.
5.	Equipment maintenance fees including computer systems, scanners, imaging systems, and software updates, etc.
6.	Annual fees for software licenses and data backup, storage and retrieval.
7.	The benefits and pitfalls of various vendor offerings and how to choose a credible vendor who offers comprehensive training and support and follows the standards for future compatibility.
8.	Viewing a live demonstration of the EHR to confirm that it meets your needs.
9.	Understanding how much customization, you might need and what it is going to cost.
10.	Having a checklist of all the important features that the group desires in an EHR and making sure that all questions, concerns and doubts are addressed.
11.	Getting written agreement among all parties involved about timelines for implementation so you can plan for the interruptions in your practice that inevitably happen.
12.	Vendors' references from practices with similar size and characteristics.
13.	Making sure your decision about which EHR to choose is not based on price alone but on how the system will fit your needs over the long term.
14.	Making sure that you have disaster recovery plan and offsite storage of the data.

an EHR is much reduced. One of the primary concerns with the ASP model is the transition or ownership of the data at the end of the term of the contract.

3. A Turnkey Solution is an EHR that is built, installed, and supplied by a vendor. It is "easily set up and is supposed to work out of the box." The vendor handles the networking, installation, training, scanning of paper files, transcription and billing, and any other service needed to provide the total practice solution. Turnkey solutions can be less expensive for a practice at the outset but they do not include any customization of the software. Many practices find that they have to customize the EHR screens to adapt them to the way in which the doctors in the practice like to work.

Most practices are able to recoup the cost of their EHR within three years and thereafter with improved efficiency, they experience a profit. However, much is dependent upon how well the group is able to integrate the system and get everyone to adopt it. Some practices have such difficulty getting all of their doctors to use the EHR they run parallel paper and electronic systems and the benefits of the implementation are lost. This can cause significant problems for the office staff because there are often inconsistencies in the two records and uncertainty as to which is correct. Even when the EHR is provided free of charge as is the VistA system developed by the Veterans Health Administration, the issue of cost is not eliminated because VistA requires extensive customization and training to be useful to the average physician.

The cost of implementing an EHR is not the only reason why doctors have universally been slow to adopt them. The culture of healthcare places a high value on the independence of individual doctors. Many seem to have an affinity for their paper charts that they can touch and feel and thus are reluctant give up. Almost all physicians have converted to practice management systems. Why so many remain inert when it comes to transitioning to EHRs is a difficult question. Part of the answer is that a typical practice management system is maintained by office staff, whereas EHRs require that a doctor be "hands on." Then there are the stories that have given EHRs a bad reputation. Some practices that have opted to install EHRs found that their investment did not lead to efficiency and better patient care, but to a nightmare of billing errors, lost information, computer downtime during office hours, and general chaos in reengineering the office around a system that is completely different from what they have been used to. Physicians hear these complaints and are put off. In the long term, however, EHRs generally result in greater efficiency, better quality of care, as well as economies and increased revenue through improved charge capture, decreased manual transcription, and easier reporting to government agencies and payers. They also are tied into pay for performance bonus incentives.

EHR Early Adopters Around the World

In the United Kingdom, close to 100% of primary care physicians' offices are paperless and most medical professionals are using an EHR. The UK National Health System program, initiated in October, 2002, set a goal that every individual

Table 2.3 Features of the NHS Care Records Service (NHS CRS)

1.	An electronic booking service (Choose and Book) – hospital or clinic appointments.
2.	Electronic Transmission of Prescriptions (ETP) – between General Practitioners (GPs), pharmacies and the Prescription Pricing Authority (PPA).
3.	The HealthSpace Web service that allows patients to access their NHS care records.
4.	The National Network (N3) – IT infrastructure and broadband connectivity for the NHS.
5.	Contact – a central e-mail and directory service for the NHS.
6.	Picture Archiving and Communications Systems (PACS) for access, storage, and retrieval of digital medical images.
7.	IT supporting primary care – Quality Management and Analysis System (QMAS – collects national achievement data, and computes the points and payment value earned by GP practices); GP2GP (enables the transfer of electronic health records among GP practices).
8.	Decision support – the electronic prescribing program; online knowledge and library systems: integrated care pathways; e-referral support; support for ordering clinical investigations; etc.
9.	The national, central database (Spine) which stores the summary patient records and also indicates where the full local records are held[5].

in the UK would have an electronic health record that could be accessed at any point of care throughout the country, including the doctor's office, hospitals, and walk-in clinics, by 2010. This project is the largest of its kind in the world, and connects over 100,000 doctors, 380,000 nurses and 50,000 other health professionals and 50 million patients. Since 2002, every individual in the United Kingdom at birth is given a 10 digit NHS unique number identifier that is included in the health record. This number is available throughout the country wherever and whenever the patient might seek care. The ambitious UK initiative also includes electronic prescribing and electronic booking of appointments. Benefits to the patient include reduction in medical-error faster treatment due to the e-record's availability and legibility; information sharing among doctors and patients; and support for clinical decision making.

The features of the NHS Care Records Service (NHS CRS) are included in Table 2.3.

In Sweden, the Netherlands, and Australia, over half of all primary care physicians are using EHRs. In Sweden, 90% of primary care physicians use it; in Denmark, the figure is 62% and in Australia 55%. These systems chiefly serve local practices and typically do not share information with other sites.[6]

Health Information Exchange and Compatibility

EHR systems have typically been built from a combination of homegrown and off the shelf software programs, making it difficult to interconnect EHRs and exchange data seamlessly. Most physicians want to be able to send and receive information directly to and from their EHR to the local hospitals, other specialists, laboratories, and pharmacies. Although a group practice may not think about exchange of information when initially considering an EHR, it will become important to them. Standards are a practical prerequisite to allowing disparate EHRs to talk to one another and exchange data. There are two industry standards that a medical practice purchasing an EHR system should be aware of: Clinical Document Architecture (CDA) that specifies how a computer program containing patient data can generate a summary document that includes a standard set of information about a given patient, and HL7 v. 3 which specifies how two different computer programs (e.g., a hospital's lab system and a physician's practice EHR system can exchange data. The HL7 standards are built around "messages" that occur in a healthcare setting like "placing an order" or "communicating a result." Most vendors' products conform to the HL7 and CDA standards, but it is important to ask those questions before considering a purchase. For seamless exchange of data, interfaces as well as built in standards are generally required. The practice that wishes to install an EHR will have to consider customization and maintenance that is over and above the initial purchase. It is important to know all the parameters.

The process for certifying that a commercial EHR product includes the necessary features that physicians and patients need for it to work properly was established by the Certification Commission for Healthcare Information Technology (CCHIT^{SM}). CCHIT was founded in 2004 by three US industry associations in healthcare information management and technology: American Health Information Management Association (AHIMA), Healthcare Information and Management Systems Society (HIMSS), and The National Alliance for Health Information Technology (Alliance) who provided initial funding. The mandate for the CCHIT is to set criteria and help to accelerate the adoption of health information technology. What these standards and certifications mean for the physician wishing to implement an EHR is that the product they are considering meets quality milestones that are important, particularly in the long term.

Regional Health Information Organizations Information Exchange

A regional health information organization is a collaborative of health plans, health care providers, and hospitals in a given geographic area that collects patient information for collation, distribution, and coordination of care. This information is stored on a secure server and is available to all providers in the collaborative, on a need to know basis, including hospital employees and physicians, whether the patient is seen in the physician's office the emergency department or in an outpatient clinic. Regional Health Information Organizations (RHIO) collaboratives are self-governing and committed to a common set of standards to facilitate interoperability and information sharing among the various medical entities.

There are several RHIOs throughout the United States – no two are exactly alike. Some have met with more success than others.

Case Study: The Indiana Network for Patient Care and Indiana Health Information Exchange

Indiana is a pioneer in regional health information exchange. Enabled by the Regenstrief Medical Records System (RMRS), the Indiana Network for Patient Care (INPC) is a sophisticated, secure wide-area network, and clinical data repository that incorporates standard vocabularies to enable data exchange from multiple, unrelated information technology systems. INPC enables healthcare professionals to view as a single virtual record all of a patient's previous care that is housed in a data repository. This electronic network provides e-mail services, electronic medical record access, medical library services and numerous special purpose functions (variously) at each institution. It also delivers clinical data to the central RMRS medical record system from a host of different departmental and administrative systems and enables care providers and researchers to have access to the RMRS.

The RMRS is a physician-designed integrated inpatient and outpatient information system that includes 30 years of data. Over 34 million physician orders have been entered into this computerized order entry system that also provides unique clinical decision support and guidelines. The RMRS has had 12 million registration events since 1972 and 12 million drug orders; 954 million numeric or coded patient observations; 22 million dictated reports; and 577,000 EKG tracings. It is accessed more than 400,000 times a month. The RMRS is used at more than 40 inpatient and outpatient facilities in Indianapolis and the surrounding counties and is the largest coded, continuously operated medical records system in the United States. Physicians and other health care providers enter information from physical examination, diagnostic images, clinical laboratory tests, and other patient treatment data at terminals located at the point of care.

One physician's experience with the Indiana Network for Patient Care illustrates why the system is efficient and effective for doctors and patients:

> *"A gentleman came into the ER with a heart attack and the normal course of treatment would have been to give him clot busters. By checking the electronic medical record available through the system I learned that the patient had recent surgery so obviously clot busters would not have been wise. Since I had all the notes from the hospital in front of me, I was able to choose a safer treatment option."*

The Indiana Health Information Exchange was formed by the Regenstrief Institute, local hospitals, and other key stakeholders to bring tools and technologies developed by the researchers at the Regenstrief Institute out to the healthcare market in Indiana. Its flagship service, called the **DOCS4DOCS®** service, is a community-based clinical messaging service that electronically delivers test results (such as laboratory, radiology) and other reports (such as transcription, admissions, discharges, and transfers) securely and efficiently to physicians through a secure online portal. Indiana Health Information Exchange (IHIE) works with hospitals, pharmacies, private laboratories, and other medical care organizations and facilities to deliver this information.

The IHIE also administers the Quality Health First™ program, a clinical quality program for health and chronic disease management. This community service combines medical and drug claims data and clinical data to provide physicians with reports, alerts, and reminders to help monitor patients' health and wellness, including the management of common, chronic diseases. The program also includes childhood immunizations and mental health screening and follow-up. Participating health insurers will also use these reports to provide meaningful incentives based primarily on the physician's high performance and significant improvement of the overall health of their patient population.

IHIE is a 501(c) (3) organization, governed by a board of directors with representatives from participating health systems, public health agencies, and physician groups. Local hospitals, other stakeholders and US Federal grants provided the initial seed money. IHIE has become self - sustaining by charging user fees to deliver results to participating hospitals, laboratories, and other major data sources. Physicians are not charged for access to the information.[7]

Case Study: The Taconic Health Information Network and Community

Taconic Health Information Network and Community (THINC) is a multistakeholder community-wide collaborative in New York's Hudson Valley. The eight county region has a population of over two million patients with over 5,000 practicing physicians. THINC is composed of a broad range of stakeholders from the public and private sectors, including physicians, hospitals, safety net providers, payers, employers, laboratories, public health authorities, quality organizations, state government representatives, community business leaders, a consumer advocacy group, and others in the healthcare industry The primary purpose of the THINC RHIO is to advance the use of health information technology through the sponsorship of a secure Health Information Exchange (HIE) network, which serves over 350,000 individuals and promotes the adoption and use of interoperable EHRs and the implementation of population health improvement activities, including public health surveillance and reporting, pay for performance, public reporting, and other quality improvement initiatives.

Over 500 physicians use the THINC RHIO health information exchange by accessing an Internet-based portal. The HIE includes all of the hospitals and 99% of the reference laboratory data in two of the eight counties in the region. It is maintained by a sustainable funding model with data transfer fees paid by the hospitals and laboratories. THINC RHIO is also overseeing the implementation of EHRs through the eight-county region. Physicians pay a subscription fee for implementation, training, and ongoing support of the systems. The collaborative provides extensive training programs to educate doctors about the capabilities of information systems, and how they will benefit their practices and their patients by enhancing safety, improving quality, and decreasing cost. Their objectives are to increase the completeness of data available to physicians at the point of care, incorporate tools for chronic care management, and facilitate process improvement in physician practices.

Dr. Mark Foster, a primary care physician who serves as the Vice Chairman of the THINC RHIO views this model as the way to save primary care medicine and the small practice model where over 80% of patients in the US receive care. This is accomplished by providing these groups with digital technology that enables them to collaborate and interconnect with others in the system. Dr. Foster, himself, worked in a paper-based practice for many years and sees the advantages of an electronic health record and the ability to exchange information with hospitals in the region. Now his patient's health records are available at any location in which he is caring for that patient. He also sees the economies and efficiencies gained by the ability to order labs for a patient and have them automatically returned to the patient's chart and the doctor's inbox through the information exchange.

THINC RHIO is constantly expanding and evolving with the addition of new technologies such as the ability for primary care doctors to link records directly to specialists. Dr. Foster contends that all of these digital technologies not only provide better quality healthcare for the patients of physicians who participate in the THINC RHIO, but also help doctors meet criteria for pay for performance incentive programs that help them to realize a financial payback.[8]

RHIOs in the United States were conceived as the initial building blocks to support a national health information infrastructure. However, not all RHIOs have been successful. When the idea of the RHIO was first introduced, there was much concern that legal barriers including fraud, abuse, antitrust, and privacy laws would prevent communities from successfully launching. However, it has turned out that the structure and financing of certain RHIOs, not the legal issues, have created impediments for those RHIOS that have had difficulties maintaining their operations. Nearly one quarter of the RHIOs known to exist in mid-2006 were defunct by early 2007. This disturbing trend indicates that establishing a nationwide information exchange that should benefit physicians and patients faces many hurdles and roadblocks.[9]

Santa Barbara Country Care Data Exchange (SBCCDE)

The Santa Barbara Country Care Data Exchange (SBCCDE), which began in 1999 to connect hospitals and doctors' offices in this California region, failed eight years later because it could not sustain itself. Once the $10 million initial grant ran out, the Santa Barbara healthcare community decided not to provide more funding to keep it going. Many of the doctors who were members of the RHIO are still using their EHRs but the dream of sharing data across practices no longer exists. One of the weak points of the SBCCDE RHIO was its desire to do everything at once – i.e., promising that all health care providers would be able to share patients X-rays, lab work, prescriptions, discharge summaries, and other data. The other problem they ran into was finding a way to provide a return on investment, especially for healthcare providers who cannot raise their fees. They simply could not find the right model.[10]

It is not only feasible and cost effective, but desirable for hospitals, pharmacies, laboratories, and clinical practices to share information, maintain it in a secure data repository, and access that data to get it to the point of care when and where it is needed. What is important for physicians to take away from these examples is that working with a larger regional healthcare organization can provide a pathway to implementing digital technology and data exchange that will result in a more efficient, cost effective, safer medical environment for physicians and patients. Taking this concept to the next level, when healthcare data exchange becomes ubiquitous, a patient who resides in Portland Oregon and has a local physician can show up in the emergency room at a New England hospital and his or her medical record and health history can be immediately accessed by those doctors in the emergency room.

This concept is predicated upon a National Health Information Infrastructure (NHII) that would be funded, with a combination of public and private dollars, and fosters the establishment of regional collaborations. The effort is similar to one initiated by the Federal government several years ago, when a visionary program set out to establish the Interstate Highway System which everyone now benefits from. Establishing the NHII would require cooperation and financing coming from several Federal, State and local health organizations, healthcare providers, health plans and purchasers, consumer and patient advocacy groups, community organizations, academic and research organizations. This is a monumental task at best and one that has been talked about extensively with little or no direct funding or action.

Computer Physician Order Entry

Every intervention in a patient's care, outside of surgery, is initiated by a physician's written order. CPOE automates that order writing process and provides a computer-based system of ordering medication and treatment for patients in the hospital setting. CPOE systems eliminate the need for transcription and improving medical documentation. Generally, CPOE software is bundled with clinical decision support software (CDSS) that can perform drug allergy checks, drug-laboratory value checks, drug–drug interaction and issue alerts and reminders helping ensure that the order does not have any clinical conflicts. Other benefits of CPOE include the elimination of repetitive testing and improved turnaround times that speed up the treatment process and shorten a patient's hospital stay.

Saint Raphael's Hospital in New Haven, Connecticut, a 511-bed acute care hospital that admits approximately 22,000 patients annually, and is affiliated with Yale Medical School, experienced a reduction in medication turnaround time from over 2 h to 18 min with CPOE. The hospital is dealing with a severe nursing shortage and the efficiencies of the CPOE system help them meet the demands of their patient load more effectively.[11]

Ohio State University Health System documented that using CPOE completely eliminated transcription errors, as there is no illegible handwriting for nurses, clerks, and pharmacists to decipher. Their studies also documented that CPOE resulted in a time reduction of 25% for laboratory orders, 43% for radiology orders, and 64% for pharmacy orders.[12]

CPOE systems are generally part of an IT solution in the hospital that seeks to reduce medical errors when handwritten prescriptions and orders for labs and tests are passed from a physician onto the nursing staff and through other staff individuals to the labs and pharmacies. Therefore, implementing CPOE is a complex process that requires extensive reengineering. That process affects everyone in the clinical setting because the changeover alters the way clinicians organize their work and take care of patients. If a CPOE implementation is to be successful, the sensible way to launch is with a detailed workflow analysis that looks at all points in the clinical process and defines current practices in the manual system. This should be diagramed in a data flow chart with the patient at the center. The next step is to do a similar data flow analysis that maps changes and demonstrates how the doctors and hospital staff will be affected by CPOE. Since the key to success is a proper system architecture that fits into the workflow of the institution, it is crucial that the IT department, CPOE vendor, clinical staff, lab technicians, and pharmacists work together to lay out the plan, reengineer workflow processes, and implement the appropriate solution.

Clinicians must be involved from the beginning discussions, if the CPOE installation is to be embraced and used properly. User education and training are important components of a successful implementation but also take time out of the busy clinician's day. Ideally, the CPOE application should be available to physicians in their offices and in their homes via a network with the hospital. Involvement in the CPOE planning process by offering financial incentives to clinicians help to convince them to embrace the systems, and learn to use them, will help the institution realize the benefits of CPOE for all the stakeholders.

Personal Health Records

"Nothing about Me without Me"

Donald Berwick MD Institute for Healthcare Improvement (IHI)

The Personal Health Record (PHR) is an electronic application used by the patients with their providers to maintain and manage health information (and that of others for whom they are authorized), in a private, secure, and confidential electronic environment. PHR digital technology makes patient data available to the patients, providers, and institutions that are involved in patient's care. PHRs mean different things to different people and exist in many configurations. They include the following:

1. A written synopsis of a patient's medical heath and history on paper – good for an emergency but not useful in a shared environment.
2. An electronic medical health and history that resides on a commercially available Web site that the patient creates and maintains, e.g. Medem's IHealth Record or the PHR that an individual can set up at WebMD that a provider may access and add to.
3. A digital electronic medical record that the patient creates that is populated by an individual, by health institutions, by providers, by payers and represents a comprehensive accounting of the patient's medical information. It is the model

upon which Microsoft Healthvault and Google are building their personal health record service.

4. A digital health record that is available from a payer (Aetna, Cigna, Blue Cross Blue Shield, etc.) and is populated with claims information.
5. The PHR on a smart card, similar to a social security card or an ATM card. The PHR smart card includes a patient's complete health history and information on individual illnesses as well as demographic and geographic information, insurance data, medication lists, healthcare providers' names and contact information, and insurance records. The patient carries the PHR smart card at all times, just like a credit card. The primary care physician has complete access to the medical information on the card. When the patient visits the PCP, the card is automatically updated with new information. Smart cards use digital signature technology with encryption and are thus more secure and private than many other forms of PHRs. In case of an emergency, the information on the smart card can be retrieved to access the patients' latest medical information. However, a smart card can only be read on a compatible smart card reader – typically not available in most doctor's offices or emergency rooms. Therefore, the smart card solution works best within a specific geography in a collaborative health organization or a group practice where card readers are available.
6. The PHR on a microchip that costs less than an ipod, plugs into a standard USB drive on the computer, and contains all of a patient's medical information. The chip reads the record into the computer and doctors anywhere in the world can download it to a screen or print it out. The information is encrypted and accessed with a password, thus protecting the data from unauthorized viewing.
7. There is also the FDA approved implantable device that can store a medical identifier in the patient's body. The device, which is the size of a grain of rice, is implanted in an arm or leg and when a scanner is passed within six inches of the implant, a medical identifier is displayed on the screen of a radio frequency identification (RFID) reader. The data on the reader points the healthcare professional to a secure Web site where the patient's identity and the name of the patient's primary care physician reside, or where the health record may reside. This approach presupposes that the facility caring for the patient has access to the Web and that the primary care physician has an electronic health record of the patient.[13]

A standalone PHR unconnected with other systems requires that the patient enter updates as needed and empowers the patient to be in charge of his or her health information. This is a logical solution for managing patient information. However, the stumbling block with the standalone PHR is that people do not want to be bothered with them and when they do have a PHR they do not keep them up to date. Of concern to the healthcare provider is also the question of who owns the data in a PHR (see Figure 2.3). There is general consensus that the individual should own the data, but the logistics of how that works between patients and providers is unclear.

Used properly, PHRs can help patients adhere to a treatment regimen prescribed by their doctors. They also assist in communicating all of the items in a patient's

Who Should Own Data Captured in Personal Health Records?

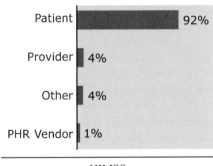

Ninety-two percent of health care IT professionals said they believe that patients should own the information stored in personal health records, while 4% said that providers should own the data. Thirty percent of respondents said they access a PHR.

HIMSS

Figure 2.3 Who should own the date captured in personal health records? © Health Information Management Systems Society (HIMSS)

history that might be missed in a face-to-face meeting between a patient and a new doctor, or a doctor that a patient might not have seen for a long time. Until recently, the medical record gatekeeper has been the PCP. However, twenty-first century patients may see many specialists. Each specialist adds new medications, new tests, new observations, and treatments.

Jane, 53, who lives in Galveston, Texas, is diagnosed with breast cancer detected on a mammogram. Her Primary Care Physician refers her to a cancer center two hours away in Austin TX for further screening. After extensive examination, the doctors there decide the best course is surgery followed by chemotherapy. Jane's PCP wants to keep abreast of her progress and the treatment plan, since it is up to her to be sure. Jane gets appropriate screenings for other cancers for which she is at high risk. Her PCP is also responsible for Jane's follow up care.

Thus while dealing with the trauma of a cancer diagnosis, Jane is instructed to collect all of her medical records including those held by her pharmacist, gynecologist, and her X-ray films that are at the local hospital. This requires that Jane navigate through the bureaucratic system to locate and copy records. Her concern is that everyone involved in her care has all the necessary information, so there would be no chance of drug interactions, unnecessary repeat tests, and healthcare decisions based on incomplete information.

Jane's PCP, a solo practitioner, uses a paper medical chart. However, she is aggressive in encouraging her patients to generate a personal health record and she works with Jane to update her PHR to include her mammogram report and images along with information already collected from her gynecologist and pharmacist. As a result Jane is able to send her comprehensive PHR to the Cancer Center. She also backs up a copy of everything on a CD that she carries with her. After her surgery, the surgeon's report goes into the PHR along with Jane's pathology report. Now, each time Jane has a new interaction with her doctors, notes are entered into her PHR that is available to her PCP. At one point in her treatment, she developed a high fever and had to go to the emergency room at the local hospital. By calling up her PHR, the doctors were able to avoid a potentially serious adverse medication interaction.[14]

The PHR is one of the axles on which future healthcare practice revolves because it empowers the patient to be in charge. This is appropriate because it is the patient (or patient's family) who knows exactly who the patient has seen, for what purpose, and what tests and treatments were recommended and implemented. It is the patient who maintains a daily check of chronic conditions such as blood sugar readings or blood pressure that can be uploaded to the PHR. It is the patient who knows all of the healthcare providers he or she is working with. It is the patient who knows not only the prescribed medications but also the over the counter drugs he or she is using regularly. A digital PHR makes it possible to track all of this. The dilemma is what forms this health record takes.

In 2008, Microsoft and Google announced that they would offer a personal health record online based on the concept that patients and participating providers would enter data into an online database including allergies, medical conditions, medical history, laboratory results to create a health record that would be kept in a private and secure environment. Microsoft's HealthVault and Google Health position their PHR as a bridge across the silos of healthcare. They have partnered with health organizations – Microsoft with Kaiser Permanente; Google with Cleveland Clinic, Beth Israel Deaconess Medical Center, and others. In these self-contained environments, the PHR will work if they get the necessary buy in from both providers and patients who have been very slow to implement any sort of electronic health record. Primary care doctors who have most of the valuable clinical information needed to populate these PHRs have been resistant in sharing this information. Patients are also reluctant. Studies by the Markel Foundation show that although people report that they are interested in PHRs, only 11% of Americans in 2008 had attempted set one up.[15]

Case Study: EMC Corporation

EMC Corporation Implements an Employee PHR

EMC Corporation, a global technology company headquartered in Hopkinton, MA, with a workforce of over 40,500 people, provides healthcare to its employees through an employer-sponsored health plan. Concerned that employee health was not where they wanted it to be, and healthcare expenditures were increasing annually, EMC launched a major initiative, to create and maintain a healthy workforce by helping employees and family members improve overall health through a meaningful, targeted Health Management Strategy. This strategy includes Healthlink, EMC's personalized Web-based health management platform that provides EMC's US-based employees and their eligible dependents with a personal health record that is populated with data from claims information and is maintained via a partnership with WebMD. This record is designed to help EMC employees and their family members effectively monitor their own health within a private, secure environment, and empower them to control their health information and have it available anytime, anywhere in the world. Employees can go to the PHR and check a diagnosis posted after a visit with their physician. They can then use the vast WebMD database to gather information on a condition or on the medications prescribed. They can add information to their personal health record access alerts and reminders and view lab information.

The PHR is an opportunity to solve the issue of how to provide health records for everyone while enabling the exchange of health information in a secure environment. Just as the individual owns an individual's financial portfolio, even if managed by an investment advisor or an institution, the PHR is a digital health database that could be owned by the individual and managed by healthcare providers who would incorporate all of the individual's health data (observations, tests, medications, health history) into the PHR. For the nearly 70% of physicians who have not yet implemented an electronic health record system into their practice, perhaps this methodology should be adopted. With the availability of the powerful tools from Microsoft, Google, WebMD, Dossia and others, the PHR could become the standard for digital health records. As standalone records that are separate from provider input, PHRs offer little by way of coordinating and elevating the quality of care. Physicians, patients, payers, and institutions that provide care must work together to find the right digital record format for a PHR that interactively lets each of these entities enter, maintain, and purge data, and use this record as the basis of care.

Key Points

1. The Electronic Health Record provides a new way for the physician to maintain records on patients addressing a myriad of problems, including lost or misplaced paper charts and missing information at the point of care, (especially for treating patients with chronic illness). The EHR facilitates the exchange of health information with hospitals, specialists, labs and pharmacies and provides the physician with decision support tools for best practices.
2. The benefits of an EHR include more accurate and timely billing practices and a better quality of medicine by enabling the physician to be more responsive to all patients more quickly. The EHR helps the physician eliminate a backlog of paper communications that occupy time. With an EHR, the physician can digitally and efficiently communicate with labs, pharmacies, and other specialists and have all necessary information in one place at one time. Physicians can also use their EHR to run reports on thousands of patients simultaneously, particularly when there are recalls or other important points of information, they must convey to their patients. Every facet of operations from scheduling to referrals to the communication of lab results is streamlined.

3. The major barriers to adoption of EHRs are financial and cultural. Return on investment takes a long time and the smaller the group practice, the more difficult the transition and the more likely that a single individual in the practice might refuse to cooperate forcing the practice to run dual systems.
4. Although the EHR is more secure than a paper chart, because it is behind a firewall and requires access authentication, security is a major concern with the digitization of information, and must be addressed.
5. EHR standards are evolving and it is important for groups investing in an EHR to understand the standards requirements that enable health information exchange.
6. RHIOs that assist healthcare stakeholders in a specific geography provide a viable way for seamless exchange of health information. However, building and sustaining a RHIO requires vision, commitment, funding, and technology expertise.
7. In the ideal digital world, a chain of RHIOs, supported by a National Health Information Infrastructure, will enable doctors to access and exchange information about a patient whenever and wherever it is needed.
8. CPOE is a new healthcare model that enables physicians to enter all their orders electronically. Not only do CPOE systems cut down on medical error but they also provide quicker, more effective care to patients and help to address chronic nursing and other staffing shortages.
9. PHRs are gaining traction as patients come to realize that they are the only ones who can truly manage their health. These empowered patients in partnership with their healthcare professionals will insure that their complete health information is available at the point of care.
10. With the personal healthcare record platforms available on the Internet, PHRs could become the model for digitization of health records. This will require cooperation among patients, physicians, payers, and healthcare institutions that must work together to make this happen.

References and Notes

1. Background on Electronic Health Records for Small Practices prepared by Andrew H Melczer PhD Vice President State Medical Society, Lesley Berkeyheiser Principal, The Clayton Group, Sue Miller JD Health Transactions.com, Mariann Yeager, Principal Emerson Strategic Group Inc., January 2005 (www.ehealthinitiative.org).
2. Cerner Power Works "Vascular Surgery Associate, P.A. Power Works EMR increases Efficiency, Improves Quality", http://cerner.com/public/Cerner
3. Survey of Electronic Medical Records Trends and Usage 2007 Medical Records Institute Inc. 2007.
4. Dr. Matthew Handley, medical director of health informatics at Group Health, Cooperative Seattle Washington.
5. www.informatics review.com/wiki/index.php/National_ Electronic_ Health_ Record_United Kingdom).
6. Joan S. Ash, PhD David W Bates, MD Msc "Factors and Forces Impacting EHR System Adoption: Report of a 2004 ACMI JAMIA Articles, October 18, 2004.

7. Dr. Marc Overhage Associate Professor of Medicine, Regenstreif Institute, Indiana University, Indianapolis, Indiana.
8. Dr. John Blair, President and CEO Taconic IPA Inc. and Dr. Mark Foster Chairman of the Board Taconic IPA Inc. and Vice Chairman THINC RHIO.
9. Julia Adler-Milstein, Andrew P. McAfee, David W. Bates, and Ashish K. Jha The State Of Regional Health Information Organizations: Current Activities And Financing Health Affairs Web Exclusive, December 11, 2007.
10. Santa Barbara Country Care Data Exchange: Lessons Learned, ihealth reports, California Healthcare Foundation, August 2007.
11. Computerized Physician Order Entry: Costs, Benefits and Challenges, January 2003 Prepared by First Consulting Group, for Federation of American Hospitals and Advancing Health in America, AHA 42.
12. Quality Patient Safety and Cost Effectiveness Through Leadership and Health Information Technology, Douglas E. Goldstein, Medical Alliances Inc p. 6, 7 www.medicalalliances.com
13. John Halamka MD. Straight from the shoulder. New England Journal of Medicine 2005; 353(4):331–333.
14. Connecting Americans to their Healthcare, Final Report, July 2004. The Markle Foundation and the Robert Wood Johnson Foundation.
15. www.cio.com/article/print/146801

Chapter 3
Communication

*The medium is the message because it is the medium that shapes and
controls the search and form of human associations and action.*

Marshall McLuhan
Understanding Media: The Extensions of Man, McGraw Hill,
New York, London 1964

The Media, the Message, and the Internet

In 1964, Marshall McLuhan, sociologist and contemporary thinker wrote in
Understanding Media: The Extensions of Man that the dominant communication
media of our time will shape the way humans think, act and ultimately perceive the
world around them. "The media are extensions of our senses; as they change, they
utterly transform our environment and affect everything we do, they "massage" or
reshape us. They are so pervasive in their personal, political, economic, aesthetic,
psychological, moral, ethical, and social consequences that they leave no part of us
untouched, unaffected, unaltered."[1]

Little did Mr. McLuhan realize the how true these words would become a short
30 years later in a world where the Internet has such a profound influence on how
people think, act and interact. The Internet has dramatically changed human communication. Most technologies take a minimum of 20 years to truly take hold and
that was true of the Internet that became a part of the everyday lives of most individuals in the 1990s. In healthcare, this cyberspace revolution has reinvented the
lives of healthcare professionals and their patients. Healthcare information is now
ubiquitous; out of the control of the physician and in the hands of all parties
involved in a healthcare situation: physician, patient, family, and other healthcare
providers. With the amount of information now available, the options that weigh in
on a single healthcare issue has increased on an order of magnitude. The consequences of this require that every healthcare team insure that each communication
encounter with a patient is efficient and meaningful.

A story reported in the Wall Street Journal (April 9, 2006) illustrates the power
of communication technology tools - scanning, email, uploading and downloading
to the Internet, CDs - to get the right information into the right hands to solve a

N.B. Finn and W.F. Bria, *Digital Communication in Medical Practice*,
DOI: 10.1007/978-1-84882-355-6_4, © Springer-Verlag London Limited 2009

serious healthcare problem. It is a poignant reminder of our vulnerability in a critical health situation, and how important it is to use every means available, to insure the life and safety of human beings.

Tengis Baasanjav was born in Ulan Bator Mongolia with a heart condition that, if untreated, is always fatal. Fortunately, Tengis had an Uncle, Soyola Baasanjav who was working in California, and a grandmother who would not give up. When Soyola received an email from his mother outlining the details about his nephew's condition, he immediately sent emails to cardiologists throughout the United States seeking help. When it seemed all but impossible to get the information about Tengis, to doctors in the U.S, Grandmother Unursaikhan Shukhert made it happen.

*Dr. Evan Garfein, a Harvard University medical resident at Boston Children's Hospital, spotted an email in his inbox, where the words **pediatric cardiologist** caught his attention. Dr. Garfein was drawn to this baby's story and brought the case to the attention of Dr. Pedro del Nido, chief of cardiology at Children's Hospital, who agreed to waive his fee and operate on the baby from Mongolia. There were hurdles before surgery could take place. Dr. del Nido needed to see an echocardiogram of the baby's heart to be sure that there were not going to be insurmountable complications. The first set of films sent by email was inadequate for a full diagnosis. With persuasion local doctors made a second set of films that they recorded on VHS tape. Sending the tape would take nine days - too long to wait. So using equipment at the University of Mongolia, arranged for by Grandmother, Unursaikhan, the local doctor, was able to upload the echocardiogram that Soyola downloaded, burned on a CD, and sent overnight to Dr Garfein. With the cooperation of several agencies that helped to fund the Baasanjav family trip to the US and cover the hospital costs, Tengis was successfully operated on. A year later he is walking around the family home, like a normal child.[2]*

The Institute of Medicine (IOM) issued a statement in 2001 that twenty-first century medicine should be "*care based on **continuous** health relationships.*" "Patients should receive care whenever they need it and in many forms, not just face-to-face visits. This ruling implies that the healthcare system should be responsive at all times - 24/7 - and that access to care should be by every possible means including email, telephone, online e-visits, and face to face encounters.[3]

Digital technology unlocks communication channels and reshapes the conduct and delivery of healthcare, to save lives and deliver better, safer medicine. Although digital communication between patients and their healthcare providers is becoming more frequent, there is a long way to go. There are three possible modes of communication for healthcare interactions: a face-to-face encounter; the telephone, and online communication including email, through portals and use of the Internet for eVisits.

The Telephone

The history of the telephone is a good example of what happens when a technology becomes widespread. The original telephones had no dial tone. To make a call the individual had to pick up the receiver and wait for an operator to come on the line.

The caller told the operator the number and the call was placed. Next came direct dial telephones that put the power of making a call directly into the hands of the user. For most people, this was a first experience interacting with a computer.[4]

In the twenty-first century practically every person on the street from London England, to Times Square in New York City, to Tokyo, Japan, to Beijing, China, is carrying a cell telephone. People spend more time each day communicating than in any other activity. Using their tiny wireless devices, individuals now access the Internet and send email and text messages, take photographs, and listen to music. In an emergency, the telephone enables a synchronous communication to address an immediate need. Ironically, health information technology had its roots in the invention of the telephone. Chief among the early subscribers of telephone service were doctors and druggists. Prior to the invention of the telephone, an individual or someone in the family had to physically go to the doctor's office to summon the doctor. Once the telephone was commercially available, a doctor did not necessarily have to make a house call or have the patient come in for a face-to-face visit. The telephone became a reliable, alternative mode of communication.

There is a downside to using the standard telephones for communication between physicians and patients. There is the age-old problem of telephone tag that can be time consuming and frustrating for patients and physicians. Telephone conversations can be interrupted; telephone messages are often overlooked, misplaced, or transcribed incorrectly.

Smart Phones and PDAs

The smart phone or the handheld device called a PDA (Personal Digital Assistant), are emerging as essential tools for the ePhysician. In this decade, the smart phone and the PDA have merged into one single handheld device that can be used by physicians as digital organizers that contain calendars, notepads, address books, and email capability, telephones, and connections to the Internet. With a PDA, a physician can access patient health records, prescribe medications, make medical calculations, code and bill for procedures, and check on the latest treatment of a complicated disease, access the Physicians Desk Reference or other drug databases from anywhere and at anytime. Using the same device, the physician can call or email patients. PDAs also facilitate patient data management and exchange between covering doctors in the hospital. They often include an audio feature that enables the clinician to dictate notes into the device that can be transcribed, or transmitted to an electronic health record, or stored and saved. Cameras built into most smart phones enable patients or clinicians to photograph and send all types of graphics digitally to a physician or to a computer that houses a patient's record. This technology convergence places more information power in the hands of the eHealth professional at the point of care and is growing at a rapid rate.

Frank suffers from sleep apnea. A Bluetooth enabled smart phone monitors Frank while he sleeps. A wireless monitor clipped to his finger or toe overnight collects data on the apnea episodes that occur during the night and sends that

Table 3.1 Smartphone Penetration Among Active U.S. Physicians (2006–2011)

	2006	2007	2008	2009	2010	2011
Penetration	49%	52%	60%	65%	68%	70%

(Defining the "Black Bag" for the twenty-first Century: The Evolution of Mobile eHealth Applications," The Diffusion Group, (a "think tank" that focuses on research new media and the digital home), located in Dallas TX.) www.tdgresearch.com

information to Frank's doctor over a cell phone. Frank and his physician analyze the information, confer over a cell phone, and decide on a treatment.

The Diffusion Group, a market research firm focused on the Connected Home and IP Media markets claims that smart phones are rapidly emerging as the "black bag" of the new millennium - an all in one diagnostic kit and communication device for the healthcare professional as well as a health information and monitoring tool for the health-conscious consumer. They predict that and the number of practicing physicians who will use internet-enabled smart phones will grow from 405,000 in 2006 to more than 612,000 by 2011 in the US (see in Table 3.1).

The specific features of hand-held devices make them well suited for the mobile twenty-first century eHealth professional. They are small, lightweight, and easy to use and handle. They automatically turn off when not in use. They are equipped with an area for managing personal information that is separate from the clinician's practice. If a patient has a chronic condition, the doctor can work out an arrangement to have the patient send their vitals from their home such as blood pressure and blood sugar and weight to the PDA. Like everything else, they have their drawbacks. The small screen, the short battery life, and rampant privacy issues still loom as obstacles. However, the availability of these tools to enable a clinician to become more proactively involved with patients and offer the continuous patient care mandated by the IOM guidelines makes this a technology that healthcare professionals cannot ignore.

Electronic Mail

Conventional email is the most common form of electronic communication and has the potential to improve both the quality and efficiency of healthcare delivery. It is inexpensive or free. It is something people throughout the world use everyday. When a group of patients were polled, more than 70% indicated that they would *"like to communicate with their doctors via email,"* but only a small percentage (under 10%) are doing this because their doctors do not use email. Many also responded that use of email would influence their choice of a doctor, if they were to change physicians. Although a very small percentage of physicians engage in email with their patients, nearly 100% say they are connected to the Internet and use email for other purposes.[5]

Mary, 42, is an accountant in a small firm 50 miles North of Madison, Wisconsin. She has high cholesterol and high blood pressure. Several days after she had her annual visit with her physician, and at the height of tax season, Mary became alarmed by a sudden spike in her blood pressure. She sent an email message to the doctor asking if she should come in immediately. The doctor wrote back within a couple of hours that she should calm down; watch the pressure; increase her medicine for a couple of days and send another email in 24 hours with the blood pressure results. The quick two-way communication enabled by email allowed Mary to be at her desk, until she heard back from the doctor and saved her from losing a day of work during a crucial time.

Email has proven that it will save unnecessary visits to the doctor's office in nonemergency situations. Because email extends care beyond the office visit, it enables patients to ask those pressing questions that they forgot to ask or did not think about, or were embarrassed to ask when they were face to face with a healthcare professional. The result is a more comfortable relationship between the physician and the patient. Dr. Eric Liederman, Medical Director of Clinical Information Systems at UC Davis Health System in California, contends that those physicians who use email find that it improves their productivity, decreases their overhead costs, and improves their patients' access to their services.

Dr. Danny Sands and Dr. Tom Delbanco thought leaders in the area of digital communications in medicine wrote in the New England Journal of Medicine in 2004: "Email is qualitatively different from all other forms of communication. It breeds informality and spawns new shorthand. It encourages short messages, permits rapid-fire interchange, and facilitates leisurely intercourse. Judging from our early experience in a practice that offers secure electronic communication, email gives doctors and patients more time to think. Doctors and patients move closer together and trust grows strikingly. Interchange becomes more personal and office visits seem more efficient and less emotionally charged."[6]

Obstacles to Email Use

Many physicians' reluctance to use email with their patients' stems from several factors:

1. Reimbursement for time - physicians fear they will be overwhelmed by the number of emails and online consults that are not currently reimbursed, at a time when they are already overscheduled and overextended. Although physicians readily admit that they are not reimbursed for the telephone calls and the telephone tag they experience with their patients, many feel that email will occupy more time than a phone call and prevent them from having the bandwidth to practice medicine properly. In reality, those physicians who are email users have found that email saves them time when they need to communicate with patients, especially for those patients who have chronic conditions that require monitoring.

2. Legal issues - physicians worry that email is a permanent written record that can be used against them in a malpractice lawsuit. They also fear that some patients willfully, others unwittingly will misuse email, creating other legal nightmares. Doctors are also concerned that a patient will use email in an emergency when it is essential that the patient call or page the doctor for help.
3. Security - physicians worry about the security/confidentiality of email exchanges via the Internet and about their liability if by chance an email gets into the hands of an unauthorized individual. There are two email configurations: email over the public Internet and secure email that goes through a patient site or portal and is protected with encryption and firewalls.

Email Benefits

There are many situations where email is the communication medium of choice:

1. Email is particularly effective in treating patients with chronic conditions such as diabetes, hypertension, congestive heart failure, etc. who send daily readings by email to their physicians. With this updated information, the doctor can regulate medications and track the patient's progress.
2. Email enables the physician to send links to groups of patients who have similar conditions.
3. Email takes real-time constraints out of noncritical doctor-patient communications and enables the doctor and patient to have an ongoing discussion to clarify all of a patient's latent issues and concerns. It also shortens the time in dealing with prescription refills.
4. Email improves continuity of patient care especially if used for previsit information gathering and postvisit follow-up for test results, scheduling of tests and for answering patient questions that they forgot or did not want to ask during the face-to-face visit.
5. Email allows the patient to send graphical images so that wounds, rashes, and other external injuries can be viewed, reviewed, and resolved.
6. Email spans geographic distance. It gives patients the comfort that no matter where in the world they might travel they can communicate with their personal physician who can connect them with local medical personnel if necessary.[7]

Deborah was on vacation in the Southwest when she injured herself climbing. She saw a local physician who diagnosed a tendon dislocation and recommended immediate surgery. Unwilling to undergo surgery in an unfamiliar hospital, she sent email to her primary care physician asking whether or not she could wait for surgery until she got home. Using email technology, her primary doctor set up a consult with an orthopedist reviewed what had happened and told her it was okay to wait. When Deborah arrived home four days later everything was in place for her surgery, which was successful.

Email Guidelines

Many of the barriers to using email are addressed when physicians set up specific guidelines that they review with their patients. These guidelines include:

1. A physician should only use email with an individual with whom the physician has an established relationship; that includes having a documented patient history and physical evaluation adequate to establish conditions and treatment plans.
2. The physician must establish a procedure to process email from patients and must communicate that procedure to the patients including:

    a. Turnaround time between receipt of an email and generation of an answer (how often email is checked and a reply is generated)
    b. Average length of message
    c. Automated out of office reply when physician is not available, including estimated date of return and instructions who to contact for immediate assistance.

3. The physician should establish guidelines as to permitted email transactions such as requesting consultations, making referrals, prescription refills, billing inquiries, answers to simple questions and concerns.
4. Patient information required on every email should include: full name, telephone number, medical or hospital number (if appropriate).
5. Physician's office information on every email should include: telephone number and address of the office, instructions on how to communicate with physician when urgent care is needed, instructions on how to schedule an appointment and disclaimer notices.
6. Language of emails should be concise and to the point.
7. Use of email should only be for standard clinical questions, nonemergencies, and in instances where the patient might be able to send a digital photo.
8. Emails that are sent for nonemergencies must not be trivial, nor should they waste the doctor's time.
9. Email should NEVER be used for:

    a. Emergencies
    b. Time sensitive requests
    c. Issues the patient wishes to be kept confidential.

10. Patients and physicians must understand that email communications will be added to the patient's medical record and represents a permanent track of what is being said. With that understood, nobody is in for any surprises.
11. It is preferable that email between physicians and patients originate from a secure Internet site and not be sent via the public Internet. That way the security issues and worries that the email will land in the wrong hands are addressed.
12. Email should not be used for communication regarding sensitive medical information such as informing a patient of a disabling disease, or information regarding sexually transmitted diseases, AIDS/HIV, mental health issues, or substance abuse discussions.

Table 3.2 Template for an Email Response to a Patient

Thank you for using our EMAIL system. This is an automatic reply to the email you just sent
    your doctor. Your email has been received and will be handled as soon as possible. If this is
    an emergency, please call 911. If you need immediate assistance but it is not an emergency,
    please call your doctor.

**PLEASE BE SURE TO INCLUDE YOUR FULL NAME, REGISTRATION NUMBER,
AND DAYTIME PHONE NUMBER IN ALL EMAILS!!**

You should receive a reply to your email within the next 2 business days. If it has been more
    than 2 days, follow up by calling your doctor's office.

For emails about prescription renewals:

Include the name and dose of the medication, how many pills you have left, the name and phone
    number of your pharmacy and your doctor's name.

For scheduling:

Use email only to confirm or cancel an appointment

For referrals:

Include information about whether or not you have seen your doctor about this condition and
    what type of specialist you would like to see (if you know), and also include how you would
    like to receive your referral form (mail to you vs. picking it up at the clinic)

For billing:

Include as much information from your bill (such as invoice number and tracking number) as possible

Thank you

The Clinic

Phone number

13. The healthcare professional needs to inform the patient that the patient is responsible for notifying the physician of any types of information the patient does not want to be sent by email.
14. The healthcare professional also needs to inform the patient that the patient is responsible for protecting his/her password or other means of access to email and that the provider is not responsible for breaches of confidentiality caused by the patient.
15. Every email communication should contain this disclaimer:

"This communication may contain information that is legally protected from unauthorized disclosure. If you are not the intended recipient, please note that dissemination, distribution or copying of this communication is strictly prohibited. If you have received this message in error, you should notify the sender immediately by telephone or by return email and delete this message from your computer."

16. Physicians need to insure that a patient's email address is never used for commercial/marketing purposes.

Portals

A patient portal is a secure Website set up by a medical institution or a clinical practice, where doctors and patients can maintain continuous two-way communications, using password protected entries, in a time and space where patient confidentiality is maintained. The backbone of the portal is a gateway that provides patients and their care team with direct access to the patient's electronic health record. As a result, patients can review their medication list, medical history, and lab test results. They can schedule appointments, request referrals, manage their own preventive services such as mammograms, and use checklists to manage chronic health issues such as asthma or diabetes. They can upload their personal health record and store it on the portal and download links to information databases that have been posted by their eHealth professionals. They can also engage in messaging with their eHealth professionals, look up answers to questions, post blood pressure and blood sugar readings, and renew prescriptions. Physicians use portals to post summaries of an office visit, pre and postsurgery and hospital release instructions, educational information, and to broadcast messages to a large panel of patients. They can also have one-on-one communications with individual patients through the portal via an "e-visit". All of these communications are automatically captured and saved in the electronic health record for continuity of care and future reference.

Although portal communications do not replace the face-to-face visit, between a physician and a patient, the use of the portal means that a patient's care is not solely dependent upon the office visit as it has been for many decades. Interactions through the portal supplement the annual or semiannual office visit, with continuous communications at the mutual convenience of the patient and the eHealth professional. Face-to-face visits, groups sessions, email and telephone communication suddenly are driven by communication that starts at the portal.

Portals can generally be accessed from anywhere in the world by logging onto the Internet and putting in the appropriate passwords. Intrusion detection software alerts portal managers in the IT department if there are unauthorized individuals trying to access information that they do not have the right to view. Although nothing is guaranteed where security is concerned, portals offer a level of security attainable today in a password-protected environment that is far more secure than general email communications via the Internet.

Case Study: Kaiser Permanente

David Lawrence, CEO of Kaiser Permanente from 1991–2001, who championed the cause of information technology for Kaiser Permanente, and for the Nation, maintains: *"You cannot practice medicine in the* 21st *Century without information technology, it is too overwhelming."*

Kaiser Permanente (KP), which is the largest integrated health plan in America, was founded in 1945 as a not-for-profit group practice prepayment program with headquarters in Oakland, CA. By the turn of the century, Kaiser was serving the health care needs of 8.6 million members. KP includes the not-for-profit Kaiser Foundation Health Plan Inc., Kaiser Foundation Hospitals and their subsidiaries and the for-profit Permanente Medical Groups. Nationwide Kaiser Permanente employs approximately 156,000 technical, administrative, and clerical employees and caregivers and more than 13,000 physicians representing all specialties.

KP HealthConnect™ is a comprehensive health information system that includes one of the most advanced electronic health records available. The development, implementation, and maintenance of KP HealthConnect™ is a multibillion dollar strategic investment that KP initiated to improve the quality of care by connecting 8.6 million patients at KP securely to their health care teams, their personal health information, and the latest medical knowledge and research. HealthConnect™ incorporates all of the separate sources of clinical information that used to reside at the physician's office, the hospital, radiology, the laboratory, and the pharmacy into a single source to eliminate the pitfalls of incomplete, missing, or unreadable charts. It provides clinicians with decision support tools to enable them to engage in best practices. My health manager, part of the KP HealthConnect™ service available to all KP members, provides critical time-saving features, including online appointment scheduling and prescription refills. In addition, users have 24/7 online access to lab test results, eligibility, and benefits information, and even their children's immunization records. With secure e-mail messaging, members can also communicate with their doctors at anytime, from any Internet connection. More than 300,000 secure e-mail messages are sent each month to Kaiser Permanente doctors and clinicians. The system also includes administrative support applications for scheduling, registration, and billing.

When a patient arrives for care in the emergency room in a hospital without an electronic health record, basic patient information is almost always not available. KP HealthConnect™ strives to ensure that Kaiser Permanente's members' records are available more than 99% of the time. In the case that the system is not available, KP HealthConnect™ has built-in backup systems and documented downtime procedures in place to ensure continuity of care.

KP HealthConnect™ has not happened without its problems. It has had significant downtime events. KP HealthConnect™ stands out as an example of how an institution can pull together health information from a variety of sources, integrate that information with the electronic health record and an individual's personal health record, enable health information exchange, and provide a communication forum where patients and clinicians are able to be in continuous contact and have access to the latest developments in modern medicine. KP HealthConnect™ moves everyone in the KP organization a giant step away from episodic crisis sick care to an information rich healthcare environment that is ongoing, available, and accessible 24/7 for safer, better care.[8]

The eVisit

When patients have questions and complaints, they typically pick up the telephone and call the doctor. After getting through the frustrating delays of telephone tag, patient and doctor often engage in a lengthy conversation during which the doctor provides basic care instructions, and suggests a prescription that the doctor then has to call into the pharmacy. Many times the doctor recommends that the patient come in for a visit. For some doctors, the communication is via email that can include graphics. Whether it is contact by telephone or email these communications between physician and patient are typically not reimbursed. That is slowly changing.

There is a new communication vehicle, the eVisit, which takes place online, and, in many cases, is reimbursed by health insurers who recognize the efficiencies and economies that eVisits accomplish. New messaging software enables a patient to log into a secure Website and fill out templates and logic-based questions which are sent to a physician who will answer this communication and enable a dialogue to take place asynchronously. These virtual visits are generally follow-up consultations and focus on minor ailments such as colds and sore throats. The eVisit is also used for periodic checkups that do not require the face-to-face interaction especially for patients with chronic conditions. Most physicians only allow an eVisit with a patient with whom the doctor has had a preexisting relationship, with at least one prior office visit within the current year.

Unfortunately twenty-first century patients seem to need to check-in more often with their physicians in this era when there are fewer doctors to go around. According to the Centers for Disease Control and Prevention, doctor visits in the United States have increased 20% in the last five years to more than 1.2 billion visits annually, while the number of doctors is falling across the country. Patients like the eVisit because they can remain at work, at home, and on their own schedules and still get the advice that they need. Physicians who use the eVisit like it because it enables them to handle less urgent patient issues and questions without having to squeeze those patients into their already tight office schedule.

Many health plans are now reimbursing doctors for the eVisit, although by early 2008 a standard COT/HCSPCS billing code for the eVisit had not been established. The average reimbursement is in the range of $50.00. Not only are the doctors paid but the eVisit saves money for the healthcare system cutting down on the number of weekend and evening emergency room episodes for patients who cannot reach a physician and feel that they need help with matters that are important to them but not emergencies. While many physicians have been resistant to an eVisit, fearing potential HIPAA violations sophisticated online messaging software has solved that problem.[9]

The eVisit is common practice at Group Health Cooperative in Seattle WA. When patients call in with nonemergency issues they are offered the option of an eVisit, rather than an office visit. Dr. Matthew Handley estimates that two thirds of calls he gets from his patients do not require an in-office visit and can be handled through an eVisit. In the "My Group Health©," secure portal, physicians can monitor and address issues via secure messaging that would otherwise take days to answer. Group Health moved all of its patients to an electronic health record in 2003, then built the My Group Health© portal and instituted the eVisit capability. The practice is paperless.

The eVisit is on the cusp of mainstream medicine. The affordable and convenient access between physicians and patients and more efficient processing of routine issues benefit both. There is also a benefit for employers by reducing absenteeism created when workers take time off to see their physician, and by saving money on health expenditures. Paul Tang, Vice President and Chief Medical Officer at the Palo Alto CA Medical Foundation, did a study that indicated that for every $1 employers invested in eVisits, they received a $4.50 return mostly in the form of savings generated from having less lost productivity.

Case Study: Medem

This Website, launched in 1999 by the American Medical Association and other medical societies, provides secure, hosted online communications services for use by physicians and other healthcare providers, with their patients for a nominal fee (a few hundred dollars annually). For the tens of thousands of physicians who have joined Medem, the service has transformed the way they connect and communicate with their patients. IHealth is a channel to engage physicians and patients in an online relationship that replaces the need for older, phone and paper-based communications and allows for online consultation in a nonemergency situation. A video resources center enables physician members to create an introductory or educational video through You Tube and place it on their Medem hosted physician practice Website. The iHealth service also encourages patients to create and maintain a personal health record, and they can schedule their appointments or refill prescriptions online.

Henry DePhillips, Chief Medical Officer of Medem, explains that over 70% of the doctors who use iHealth have not made an investment in electronic medical records. They share access to the personal health record with their patient that becomes a virtual electronic health record. Both the doctor and the patient can add information to the PHR, so that it is completely up to date. IHealth also includes access to an extensive medical library that covers medical conditions, adherence programs, disease and treatment options, and many other issues that the doctor or the patient might need to research. Information and articles in the library are peer reviewed by members of Medem's 50 sponsoring medical societies.

With the current pay for performance incentives that health plans are offering doctors who have electronic records or online visits with patients, and the premium discounts that some medical liability carriers are offering to physicians who use the iHealth Service, a physician membership with iHealth can effectively turn into a revenue opportunity rather than a cost center, a win-win for everyone involved.

Case Study: Relay Health

RelayHealth is another widely used patient and physician asynchronous online communication and connectivity solution. Launched in 1999, RelayHealth of Atlanta, now part of McKesson Corporation, provides secure Web-enabled communications that offers patients more convenient access to their physician and connects patients, providers, pharmacies, and payers. It includes reimbursable web-Visit® consultations, prescription refills and renewals, results delivery, requests for appointment scheduling and referrals, health education information and more.

RelayHealth's webVisit® is a clinically structured Web-based interview to communicate nonurgent routine symptoms to the physician. Created by clinicians for handling online clinical questions, the formalized questionnaire template invites patients to choose from a menu of nonemergent symptoms and answer a series of questions related to that specific condition. The physician is presented with the full information to make informed quality care decisions. The doctor can access the patient's condition and respond online, by phone, or if necessary request an in-office visit. The RelayHealth system checks the patient's insurance eligibility during the webVisit®, sends a claim to the health plan for reimbursement, collects the copay and sends it to the physician. This "virtual house call" is an easy convenient and efficient way for patients to exchange information with their doctor, with the goal of improving patient care and satisfaction, enhancing relations and making healthcare more accessible to patients. The RelayHealth service requires a sign-in ID and password and can only be accessed by registered users. Patients using the service can view an audit trail detailing who has accessed their personal health record. All interactions are stored securely behind dual firewalls and encrypted prior to transmission.

Physician users of RelayHealth pay a nominal monthly fee and offer this service free to their patients who can opt to enroll to request appointments and referrals, look at the results of lab tests, refill prescriptions, engage in secure email messaging with their physicians and participate in the webVisit®. Interactive sessions are for nonurgent medical issues only, and safeguards in the form of frequent visual cues remind patients not to use it for urgent symptoms. Many of the popular commercial electronic medical records are compatible with the RelayHealth software, enabling the doctor to connect their EHR with the PHR for a more comprehensive patient record. A major benefit of RelayHealth to the physician is a reduction in the number of telephone calls for which physicians are not paid. Use of RelayHealth frees staff time to do other tasks. Doctors can send secure email blasts to target patient populations.

Charles Cutler, M.D., Chief Medical Officer for Aetna National Accounts, endorses RelayHealth as a technology that makes it easier for physicians to do business. "It facilitates communications between physicians and their patients, and helps improve patient safety. For many doctors, the ability to discuss nonemergency conditions online with their patients can save time and money."

The eVisit helps physicians, patients, hospitals, health systems, health plans, and employers insure that a continuum of care is maintained. It offers patients an alternative communication pathway to resolve nonemergency issues. In England, Chelsea and Westminster Hospitals in London have deployed an online service where patients' link to a Website affiliated with a private Internet-based healthcare provider who offers them a consult and prescribes medication. This always-available service is part of the National Health Service. As physicians become accustomed to the many ways that new technology can help them save time and money and help their patients access healthcare resources when they need them, they will more fully embrace the eVisit as another way of fostering better communication.

Key Points

1. Continuous care-based relationships between physicians and patients are essential for safe, efficient healthcare delivery. Physicians today must use all of the communication tools at their disposal to establish that level of care.
2. The telephone no longer serves as the only viable communication vehicle for physicians who need to answer questions and requests from patients. Too often telephone tag causes delays that are frustrating and patients finally give up or seek assistance from a walk-in clinic.
3. Smart phones or other personal digital assistants are essential tools for the twenty-first century mobile healthcare professional who needs instant access to medical databases, patients' electronic health records, scheduling calendars, and email messaging.
4. Patients want their healthcare professionals to use email to communicate with them and those individuals who have been using email find that it is more efficient for the physician and fosters a more satisfied patient. It also provides a communication pathway for patients with chronic conditions to keep in touch for better, safer care.
5. Email sent through the Internet clearly is not secure and privacy issues surface. Therefore, physicians should set up secure Websites where they can communicate with patients using a secure email system. Additionally, healthcare professionals need to establish email guidelines regarding how quickly a patient should expect a response; what the general content of the email might be; when to use email vs. the telephone or pagers, and parameters regarding privacy of their communications.
6. Patient portals, secure Websites initiated by a medical institution or clinical practice, are locations on the Web where patients and their healthcare professionals can communicate asynchronously via email or through an eVisit, using scripted forms and templates. On many portals patients can also schedule appointments, request referrals, manage their own preventive services, upload a personal health record, and view lab and procedure results.
7. Physicians can use portals to send blast email messages to a group of patients. Some portals include databases of best practices and clinical decisions support tools as well as the capability to feed lab results directly into an electronic health record. On some portals, physicians can send claims and billing information directly to the insurance provider.
8. The eVisit enhances physician/patient communication by enabling patients to use new messaging software to log onto a secure Website and fill out a template form that is sent to the physician who can answer the patient's concerns and

engage in an asynchronous dialogue. It is used chiefly for patients with whom the doctor has a preexisting relationship and has seen in the office. Many health plans now reimburse doctors for eVisits.

References and Notes

1. McLuhan Marshall, Understanding Media: The Extensions of Man, (The MIT Press Cambridge London, England) 1964, 26.
2. The Wall Street Journal, April 8–9 2006, "Journey of the Heart: A Boston doctor struggled to save a Mongolian boy by learning philanthropic medicine" by Ron Winslow in Boston and Mei Fong in Ulan Bator, Mongolia. Excerpt with permission from The Wall Street Journal, Copyright Clearing House
3. Crossing the Quality Chasm a New Health System for the 21st Century, Institute of Medicine, National Academy Press, Washington D.C. 2001.
4. Michael Crichton, Electronic Life How to Think About Computers, Alfred A. Knopf, New York, 1983.
5. Moyer CA, Stern DT, Dobias KS, Cox DT, Katz SJ. Bridging the electronic divide: patient and provider perspectives of e-mail communication in primary care. *Am J Manag Care.* 2002;8(5):427–433.
6. Delbanco T, Sands DZ. Electrons in flight - e-mail between doctors and patients. *New England Journal of Medicine.* 2004;350(17):1705–1707.
7. Patt MR, Houston TK, Jenckes MW, Sands DZ, Ford DE. Doctors who are using email with their patients: a qualitative exploration. *Journal of Medical Internet Research.* 2003;5(2):e9.
8. Based upon interview with Andy M. Wiesenthal, Md SM, Associate Executive Director, The Permanente Federation
9. Chuck Kilo, Greenfield Health, Portland OR 2004.

Chapter 4
Telemedicine

On November 21, 2004, eighteen-month-old baby Kate was critically injured in a car accident. She was rushed by paramedics to the closest hospital in Douglas AZ, a small rural town. When she arrived at the Douglas emergency room, Kate was in shock and minutes away from death, having lost almost two-thirds of her blood from multiple injuries. The doctor saw immediately that he would need assistance and called the closest trauma center, University Medical Center's (UMC) Level 1 in Tucson, 100 miles away. Using the Arizona Telemedicine Program (ATP) network, a trauma surgeon at UMC was able to see and examine Kate. He reviewed her vital signs, X-rays and lab tests results and virtually led the doctors and nurses in Douglas through emergency medical procedures. Once Kate was resuscitated and stabilized, she was transported to UMC for further treatment. She fully recovered.[1]

Why Telemedicine?

Telemedicine (also synonymous with teleHealth) is defined by the Institute of Medicine as "the use of electronic and communications technologies to provide and support health care when distance separates the participants." In the first decade of the twenty-first century, it is estimated by the American Medical Association that there are more than 35 million Americans who live in medically underserved areas, and it would take 16,000 additional doctors nationwide to provide services to them. As the baby boomers age and the number of medical school graduates going into primary care medicine declines, these numbers will grow. There is research that confirms that an individual of any age, who lives in a remote part of the country, is twice as likely to die from a serious injury or automobile accident as an individual in an urban area who has access to a large urban emergency department and specialized trauma care within minutes of an accident or injury. In both urban and rural communities, there is a growing population of senior citizens as well as other individuals who have illnesses and disabilities that keep them closely tied to their homes. With these population demographics and the physician and nurse shortages, the solution to providing these individuals with comprehensive health services is telemedicine.

N.B. Finn and W.F. Bria, *Digital Communication in Medical Practice*,
DOI: 10.1007/978-1-84882-355-6_5, © Springer-Verlag London Limited 2009

Telemedicine Technologies and Infrastructure

Telemedicine uses electronic information carried via telecommunications networks that include videoconferencing, Internet-enabled messaging, store-and-forward imaging, streaming media, and terrestrial and wireless communications, for example, enabling a patient at a remote clinic in South Dakota over a computer-linked interactive video system to have a leg wound examined by a world-renowned specialist in St. Paul Minnesota who is also viewing the patient's X-rays that have been sent via the Internet.

There are several facets to setting up a telemedicine network. Not every network includes all of these. They are:

1. **A hub and spoke integrated network system** that uses high-speed lines or the Internet for telecommunication links to connect tertiary care hospitals and clinics with outlying clinics and community health centers.
2. **Web browsers** that provide ease of access to information under field conditions using a wide variety of computer equipment.
3. **Point-to-point connections** to independent medical service providers at ambulatory care sites using private networks to deliver services directly or through outsourced specialty services.
4. **Single line phone-video systems** for interactive clinical consultations to provide home healthcare that connects primary care providers, specialists, and home health nurses with patients.
5. **Direct patient to monitoring center telephone links** for pacemaker, cardiac, pulmonary or fetal monitoring and related services.
6. **Web-based eHealth patient service sites** for direct consumer outreach and services over the Internet.[2]

There are also six modes for delivery of Telemedicine services. They include:

1. **Live, *real time synchronous* transmission** using interactive video, video conferencing, and the Internet, diagnostic information is collected and transmitted. A consulting physician participates in a real-time examination of the patient to render a diagnosis, treatment plan, prescription or advice. This might involve patients located at a remote clinic, a physician's office or in the home and could be used for seeking the advice of super-specialists. Labs, X-rays photos, and readings of vitals are sent ahead. An interactive conference enables the specialist to see, hear, examine, and question patients who can respond and ask questions.
2. **Store and forward asynchronous transmission**, where images or data are transferred within a building, between two buildings, in the same city, or hundreds or thousands of miles to anywhere in the world. This application can be used in a situation where a radio link between an EMT on the road and emergency medical personnel in a trauma center is established to advise the EMT on how to keep patients stable and alive before they are transported.

3. **Home monitoring** where individuals with chronic conditions such as diabetes, hypertension, and pulmonary issues use telephones, Web cams, and other monitoring medical devices that transmit images of their skin, eyes, facial expressions, and vitals to trained nurses at a remote location, who review their condition and provide the necessary advice to the patient or triage their problem to a PCP or specialist, when necessary.

4. **Online Second Opinions** is ideal for patients facing life-altering diagnoses, especially useful for patients with cancer, or patients facing surgery, where treatment options can vary. This use of telemedicine enables an individual via an interactive video hookup, to hear an opinion from a specialist who can confirm a diagnosis or offer alternative treatment plans. Many companies have incorporated online second opinion consults into their employee benefit package.

5. **Online Real Time assistance** where super specialists monitor a surgery by a local physician; or a surgery where robotic instruments hooked to cameras that are monitored by distant specialists enable local clinicians to standby as the robots perform the surgery.

6. **The eICU®** where doctors are able to watch over many intensive care units at the same time from a remote site.

One of the major benefits of telemedicine has been to reduce the number of patient visits and transfers from nursing homes, correctional facilities, and local hospitals to major trauma centers. Up to 50% of the 4,516 emergency facilities in the United States have difficulty providing at least one type of physician specialty for consultations. As a result, when rapid diagnosis and treatment is linked to outcome, patients are often transferred from one ER to another. Telemedicine enables these consultations to take place at the nursing home or in the correctional facility saving time and money and providing better care.[3]

Obstacles

Telemedicine faces a number of hurdles preventing the technology from becoming more ubiquitous. These obstacles include cost; how clinicians are reimbursed for telemedicine encounters; physician licensure; cultural barriers related to physician acceptance and technology issues, particularly the need for standards that regulate the transmission of information.

Cost

If telemedicine is to expand and reach its potential to provide high quality health services to all citizens in remote areas and to homebound individuals in urban centers, it must be done in a way that is affordable for users and feasible for healthcare providers and payers. Common practice in setting up a telemedicine network has been to use public telecommunications networks that, with deregulation, charge prohibitively high prices, particularly for high bandwidth applications like interactive video. For example, the Deaconess Medical Center telemedicine project, based in Billings Montana, spends upwards of $13,000 per month for a dedicated T-1 network with eight telemedicine sites. There are also many large areas where telemedicine services are not available that will require development and implementation of infrastructure, programs, and services. In urban areas, where there are available home health services, there are payment issues that prevent those services from reaching the people most in need. These cost issues need to be addressed through legislation and through private and public collaboration. In the longer term, they will pay back in better health and fewer emergency rooms visits for all citizens affected.

Reimbursement Policies

Medicare reimbursement policies for telemedicine are the overriding reason why this digital technology is not more widespread. Without assurance of reimbursement, many medical professionals are reluctant to consider telemedicine. In 1997 the 105th Congress passed the Balanced Budget Act of 1997 (BBA). Among numerous other Medicare and rural health care provisions was language that mandated Medicare reimbursement for interactive telemedicine care, only for beneficiaries who are treated in rural Health Practice Shortage Areas (HPSAs). HPSAs are regions that have a shortage of primary care physicians, dentists, and/or mental health care practitioners. The referring health care practitioner and the teleconsultation must originate from the designated rural HPSA. The legislation specifically includes only interactive encounters and excludes store-and-forward modes of telemedicine from being used. The reimbursement is 75% of the rate of an in-person consultation, not at the full rate that the doctor would normally charge. CMS regulations permit a physician assistant, nurse practitioner, clinical nurse specialist (MSN or equivalent), nurse anesthetist, anesthesiologist, nurse-midwife, social worker, or clinical psychologist to present the patient. Registered nurses, as well as other allied health staff, are not included on the list of eligible presenters despite their qualifications.[4]

CMS also allows reimbursement for telemedicine applications at the discretion of individual State healthcare agencies, when they prove to be a more cost-effective alternative than the traditional face-to-face consultation or examination. State Medicaid programs vary greatly in whether and how they provide telemedicine services, including differences in:

What is covered - diagnoses, procedures, second opinions
Who is covered - physician, nurse practitioner, nursing assistant, or other clinician

Which site is reimbursed - the hub or the remote site or both

Whether the physician reimbursed is licensed in that state or not[5]

This approach is uneven and does not address reimbursement for much needed home health assistance for urban residents. It ignores the plight of millions of senior citizens and disabled individuals for whom leaving the home to have their blood pressure or blood sugars monitored or a wound checked is a real hardship. As recently as 1997, home health spending was 9% of Medicare's benefit payments. That amount has declined since 1997 and in 2006, the home health benefit accounted for only 3.5% of total Medicare spending. These numbers continue to baffle since pilot studies definitively show that payment for home monitoring saves money and in urban areas significantly decreases the number of emergency room visits, which are very costly to the healthcare system.

An innovative home care program for patients with chronic obstructive pulmonary disease (COPD) that was tested in Connecticut found significant cost savings by providing more comprehensive home care services to COPD patients who previously required frequent hospitalizations. Monthly costs for hospitalizations, emergency room visits, and home care fell from $2,836 per patient before the intervention to $2,508 per patient -a net savings of $328 per patient per month.[6]

The impact of intensive home care monitoring on the morbidity rates of elderly patients with congestive heart failure was the focus of another study. The study found that with intensive home care surveillance, the total hospitalization rate dropped from 3.2 admissions per year to 1.2 admissions per year and the length of stay decreased from 26 days per year to six days per year. Cardiovascular admissions declined from 2.9 admissions per year to 0.8 admissions per year and length of stay decreased from 23 days per year to four days per year. An in-home program also resulted in significant functional status improvement in elderly patients with congestive heart failure.[7]

Licensing of Medical Professionals

The licensing process of medical clinicians and physicians in the US also inhibits the practice of telemedicine. A State Board typically licenses physicians to practice medicine. Out-of-state practice of medicine without a license is prohibited. Therefore, whether a physician is treating a patient in person or from a distant location, going beyond state lines is not allowed. State boards have denied requests from out-of-state psychiatrists, for example, to conduct therapy with their patients located in another state via telephone or videoconferencing. With the increasing sophistication of telemedicine networks, and the proven value of telemedicine to underserved and isolated patients, a legislative review governing these state restrictions is long overdue. In an era when controlling costs and healthcare professional shortages limit the physical ability of the industry to provide adequate care to everyone, legislation is needed to ameliorate this situation that restricts doctors from delivering the best care regardless of state, national, or international borders. Clearly physicians need to be licensed, but if they are in good standing there should be ways to enable these physicians to participate in telemedicine services across state borders.

Cultural Barriers

Telemedicine projects have faced the same problems inherent in introducing any new system. A certain amount of reengineering of old habits and practices must take place. Installation of the necessary equipment and applying it to how care is delivered is only the first step. Training nurses, physicians, and billing clerks is critical to a successful telemedicine network. Educating patients to accept and use telemedicine instead of depending upon traditional face-to-face interactions with healthcare providers is also critical.

Standards

Telemedicine has benefited from technical standards developed for related markets. For example, the use of ANSI H.32 × set of standards has facilitated wide-scale videoconferencing interoperability that is leading to continued growth in that market, a steep decline in the cost of equipment and the ability to conduct interactions between parties independent of the particular hardware used. In addition the development of HL7 and DICOM standards has been of great benefit especially for rapidly expanding applications in such areas as *teledermatology*. There are also about 200 *tele de facto* standards that enable telemedicine although there is more work to be done, including:

1. The Web browser driven by Hypertext Markup Language (HTML) that provides a nearly universal vehicle for presentation of information.
2. De facto technical computing standards including standard internet technology such as TCP/IP.
3. The growing body of how-to guides describe best practices for photography techniques that enable store-and-forward dermatology, effective presentation of patients during real time telemedicine consults, and other similar procedures.

Telemonitoring and Home Healthcare

As you step onto the bathmat after your morning shower, a scale woven into the fabric of your mat automatically sends your weight to a small box near your telephone. A ring on your finger checks your heart rate and oxygen level and sends this information to the box. Midmorning, a pill container you should have opened at breakfast begins to chime. Around noon, the data box near your phone sends its stored information to your doctor's office. A computer crunches the numbers and flags a sudden weight gain, a tip off that you may be in trouble. The nurse in charge of your care calls you, using a two-way video connection. A camera located in your home and one at her office enables you to see each other as you talk. You tell her you are not out of breath nor do you have other worrisome symptoms. You hold an electronic stethoscope to your chest and she listens to your heart and lungs. Together you decide that the weight gain was probably the result of too much salt in your dinner. You take an extra water pill and try to be more careful about your diet to put you back on track.[8]

This may seem far out but it is more real than fiction. The wonders of telemedicine have no limits and most of the technology is in place to transform these wonders into an everyday reality for homebound seniors and physically disabled individuals. At the beginning of the twenty-first century, one out of every eight individuals was over the age of 65 in the United States. By the year 2030 that number will double, accounting for 25% of the population. Today, one-third of the American population are the baby boomers who face the double challenge of caring for elderly parents, while dealing with their own emerging health problems as they approach retirement. With the shortage of doctors and nurses in America, the only way these millions of individuals are able to help their elderly parents, themselves, and their children is with the assistance of telemedicine.

There is no shortage of medical devices for Telemonitoring in the home. Table 4.1 lists examples of available devices.

Table 4.1 Medical Devices for Telemonitoring in the Home

1. Glucose meters that store and transmit multiple measurements to a data management system at the doctor's office and allow the medical professionals to identify trends, and track historical readings that ensure a patient's blood glucose is within their ideal range
2. Blood Pressure Monitors that allow patients to measure their blood pressure and heart rate and transmit it over the telephone
3. The Pulse Oximeter that provides immediate, reliable readings of oxygen saturation levels for patients with asthma and COPD
4. Scales of various types that measure weight and send the measurements directly to a doctor's electronic record or to a computer
5. Electronic stethoscopes that enable doctors to listen to a patient's heart from a great distance
6. Fiber optic scopes fitted with mini-cameras to examine patients' ears eyes and mouths
7. Implantable defibrillators that notify doctors when the patient experiences a potentially dangerous abnormal heart rhythm
8. Cell phones that from a pricked finger of a diabetic send information to a doctor
9. Clothing that take a continuous video of the heart's electrical activity, blood pressure, oxygen level, and other health indicators and transmit that information to a nurse at another location
10. Rings and watches that measure body temperature, heart rate, and oxygen level in the blood and send this information to a cell phone or computer
11. Bedroom floor sensors that can discern an elderly patient's unsteady gait or and potentially could predict the onset of Parkinson's disease or other neurological disorders

George is a 72-year old Air Force 78 veteran who used to rush to the veterans hospital in West Haven, CT, as many as 10 times a month for crises caused by multiple diseases including diabetes, multiple sclerosis, and advanced heart disease. Today George manages much of his care from a computer in his home that measures his blood sugar, heart rhythms, and blood pressure daily, and lets him and a Veterans Affairs nurse know if anything is wrong. In 2000, he was hospitalized four times. Today if there's a problem he can't handle by adjusting his diet or exercise, he meets with a doctor via live video, through a telemedicine system provided by the Veterans Administration.[9]

In a novel telemedicine application, Partners Telemedicine, a division of Partners Healthcare has experimented with an "orb" - a desktop glass ball that can be set to glow different colors based on preprogrammed instructions. The Orb used in conjunction with a smart pillbox helps patients adhere to their schedule of taking medications by sending a signal from the pillbox to the orb that changes color from red to green when a patient has accessed the pillbox for medication.[10]

Telemedicine for Patients in Remote Areas

TeleHealth implementations have existed in various forms since as early as the 1950s when the Nebraska Psychiatric Institute used closed circuit television to monitor patients remotely. In the twenty-first century, there are many asthmatic children in the US, who live in the Dakotas, Idaho, Montana, Oregon, Washington and Wyoming, who use Web cams in their homes to send videos to pulmonary specialists located in major medical centers that show how they are using inhalers and airflow measurement devices. If they need instructions, there are medical professionals on video to show them. There are other seriously ill children and adults who are examined and treated in real-time from local emergency rooms by critical care physicians at major medical centers. Diabetic patients on Indian reservations in rural Arizona have their retinas screened remotely by specialty doctors at the world-renowned eye centers throughout the United States for degenerative diseases that could lead to blindness.

Case Study: Hayes Medical Center

Baby James is born at the Hays Medical Center in Kansas with a suspected heart problem that requires a consult over the telemedicine network with a pediatric cardiologist. Within moments of birth, James is checked by a heart specialist, located 270 miles away in Kansas City. This doctor is able to see James, assess his skin color and respiratory effort, listen to his heart and lungs with an electronic stethoscope, review his EKG and chest X-ray, and work with a local technician to do an Echo exam. The distance that separates James from the specialist does not impede the diagnostic assessment. It is determined that James can remain in the local community. Prior to the implementation of telemedicine at Hays, James would have been transported across the state to the University of Kansas Medical Center, at considerable risk.

Hays Medical Center is located in Hays, Kansas a town of 20,000. The Center serves as a Rural Tertiary Medical Center for Northwest Kansas. Clinical Telemedicine services have connected Hays with the University of Kansas Medical Center sites in Kansas City and Wichita since 1988. Services are delivered by specialists in pediatric subspecialties of cardiology, rheumatology, neurology, and psychiatry. An oncology and hematology service for adults is staffed by a medical school faculty member who travels to Hays twice a month to see patients. These specialists also sees patients electronically twice a month. Home visits to patients with chronic diseases, along with telemedicine have resulted in a 20% reduction in hospitalizations and visits to the Emergency Department. Hays radiologists provide teleradiology services to 12 outlying communities in Northwest Kansas on a 24/7 basis. Hays has also implemented the EICU® where intensive care physicians and nurses from the St Luke's Health System in Kansas City electronically monitor all of Hays' intensive care patients from noon each day until 7 am the next morning. Fewer complications and a shortened stay in the ICU for Hays' patients have resulted.[11]

Case Study: St. Alexius Telecare Network of North Dakota

Bob is a farmer who lives in rural Minnesota. He was severely burned on his hands, chest, and back while fixing farm machinery. He was treated initially in a local hospital and after he was stable was transferred to the Regional Burn Center in Rochester, MN - 450 miles from his home. Once he was released, Bob arranged for his follow up care to be handled over the St. Alexius TeleCare network of North Dakota. He experienced three telemedicine visits each lasting 30 min, avoiding a two-day trip that would have necessitated leaving the farm with no one in charge during harvest time.[12]

Telemedicine at St. Alexius enabled Bob to keep the farm going while adhering to the treatment that his doctors felt was necessary. It provided relief to the family because they did not have to transport him 450 miles and back. St Alexius is a full service hospital with 48 hospital locations, throughout North Dakota, as well as one clinic and one nursing home. Their telemedicine network has been functioning for 10 years and enables doctors to see patients who would otherwise not be served by specialists and in some cases not even by primary care physicians. Using the network, St. Alexius doctors' conduct between 400 and 500 consults every year. Much of the work they do includes postoperative and posttrauma care. For example, they are able to check incisions of patients at home, using an otoscope. They offer speech therapy to stroke patients, conduct diabetes and Alzheimer support groups, and provide mental health services that would be unavailable otherwise.

There are occasions when telemedicine offers nontraditional services to provide care and comfort. *Joan was in the Intensive Care Unit of St. Alexius being treated for heart problems when her husband of 50 years died. The doctors at St. Alexius used the telemedicine network to connect Joan to the church so she was able to be present at her husband's funeral, giving her and the family much comfort.*[13]

Telerehabilitation

Telerehabilitation is the clinical application of consultative, preventative, diagnostic, and therapeutic services via two-way interactive telecommunication technology. Using Webcams for videoconferencing over telephone lines, videophones, and Webpages containing rich Iinternet applications, the visual nature of Telerehabilitation technology provides individuals who cannot leave their homes, or local areas with the ability to have their physical, occupational, speech and language therapy, and hearing assessments accomplished through telemedicine networks. The Veterans Administration is relatively active in using telemedicine for individuals with disabilities. They conduct several programs that provide annual physical exams, monitoring and telerehabilitation consults for veterans with spinal cord injuries.

Speech and Language Therapy

The clinical services provided by speech-language pathology readily lend themselves to telerehabilitation, because of their emphasis on auditory and visual communication. Applications have been developed to assess and treat adult speech and language disorders, stuttering, voice disorders, speech disorders in children, and swallowing dysfunction. The technology to enable these services ranges from the simple telephone to the use of dedicated Internet-based videoconferencing systems.[14]

It was a typical spring day on May 27th for Wes who worked at a National Guard Camp in North Dakota. While using a Bobcat, Wes collapsed and was taken to the local Carrington Health Center where he was diagnosed with a ruptured brain aneurysm. He was immediately flown to Fargo North Dakota where doctors were able to keep Wes alive without surgery. After 17 days in the hospital and another 27 days in rehab, Wes was able to return home. Doctors recommended that he continue with physical therapy, occupational therapy, and speech therapy. However, speech therapy was not available at Carrington Health Center near his home. A telemedicine connection from St. Alexius Medical Center enabled Wes to have speech therapy to help him swallow, eat regular food, and to speak again. Wes returned to full-time work one year after his collapse. He would not have been able to continue work at all, without the therapy.[15]

Physical Therapy

For individuals who have been injured and need physical therapy, there are three models for providing these services:

1. Teleconferencing, a live synchronous situation with the therapist and the patient communicating online via a video feed, enabling the therapist to guide the patient through various activities.
2. Virtual therapy where a patient uses reality games to assist with therapy. For example, for a patient undergoing intensive, sometimes painful physical therapy, the therapist might use a skiing game that focuses on cooling sensations to take the patient's mind off the discomfort of stretching tight muscles.
3. Web-based interactive home exercise programs where the therapist downloads specific video exercise clips and monitors the patient via a webcam or over videoconferencing. The therapist will make notes on the number of reps and frequency and work with the patient to increase the duration and intensity of the exercise, as well as to demonstrate the wrong way of doing an exercise.

At Integris Health in Oklahoma: A 25-year-old woman suffered a brain injury and was in a rehabilitation center. Insurance ran out and she was discharged to her home. The family felt unable to care for her without help. They were introduced to physical therapy telerehabilitation. Using phone connections and cameras, a physical therapist was able to teach the family to work with their daughter and help her learn how to move about. At the beginning of the teletherapy the patient could not sit in a wheelchair without assistance. At the end of 12 weeks, she was walking around the home with little assistance and able to do many things for herself.

Mental Health Services

Mental Health is one of the areas with the highest population of underserved individuals. By using a telemedicine network that enables a counselor to be in direct contact with the patient, many concerning mental health issues can be addressed.

A woman whose husband left her destitute with four children to support was in a depressed state. A local physician and nurse connected to the Rural Arkansas Delta Integrated TeleHealth system in Little Rock were contacted and arranged for a mental health consultation with a University of Arkansas psychologist. With limited income and no phone or transportation, the local police pitched in to transport this woman to a clinic where she was able to receive her teleHealth consultations with the psychologist over interactive video equipment. With this counseling, the woman was able to function and take care of her children.[16]

Telehospice: Death with Dignity

Hospice administers many health and comfort care services to patients who are nearing the end of life, including: pain management, spiritual counseling, helping people get their paperwork in order and providing reassurance to the family. The availability of telemonitoring workstations that are used to home monitor ill patients enable these individuals to transition to telehospice care as they approach death. These tools enable hospice caregivers to overcome geographic barriers and boundaries. Doctors who are concerned about the need to personally see an individual whose condition is extremely fragile but who lives a great distance away can do a virtual live examination that provides comfort and reassurance to both patient and physician.[17]

Telemedicine around the World

At Massachusetts General Hospital in Boston, doctors at the Center for Connected Health provide long distance care to patients in remote areas throughout the world and deliver cutting edge services that assist people in their homes manage and monitor their chronic illness. Dr. Joseph Kvedar, founder of the Center for Connected Health, advocates that the purpose of telemedicine is to "bring care to the patient where the patient is and when the patient needs it." The Center carries out this plan worldwide.

Since 2001, Operation Village Health has enabled physicians at the Center for Connected Health to support Cambodian health workers caring for patients at a health center in the village of Rovieng. In 2003, the program expanded to include a referral hospital in the town of Banlung - the provincial capital of the Ratanakiri province. At each of these sites, point-of-care clinical data (medical history, physical exam, labs, and digital images) are gathered by Cambodian health workers caring for patients locally. Data from select cases are emailed to volunteer physicians in Boston and in Phnom Penh for review, and within hours, recommendations are returned, allowing these isolated clinicians to not only learn from some of the best physicians in the world, but to deliver improved care to these underserved regions of Cambodia. Additional resources in the village of Rovieng include a basic point-of-care laboratory (Lab-In-A-Box) and simple clinical guidelines for the most commonly encountered medical problems. Operation Village Health has handled over 1,000 patient encounters since it was established.

The eICU: Remote Monitoring for Intensive Care

Patients, who are unlucky enough to land in Intensive Care, have cause for concern. With a severe shortage of ICU (intensive Care Unit) specialists, the expertise that an intensivist brings to the critical care unit is missing in many hospitals. Less than 6,000 Intensivists are actively practicing in the US, leaving only 13% of ICU patients receiving dedicated intensivist care. With the aging population and its anticipated need for intensive care, the acute shortage of specialists compounds the problem. When an intensive care doctor is available to manage the ICU, studies show that a patient's chance of dying in the ICU decreases by 30%.

Two creative physician-entrepreneurs from Johns Hopkins, in 1998, founded a company called ViSICU, using telemedicine technology to address this problem. They created the eICU®, a central command room outfitted with cameras that beam directly to each patient's bedside. Broadband technologies and land-based wireless networks allow continuous communication of data, voice, and video at ultra high speeds. The eICU® can be located within a hospital complex or off site at a completely different location minutes or miles from the intensive care unit. It is manned 24/7 by intensive care doctors and nurses. All of the information that the doctor needs to make a decision comes directly into the eICU®. From a control station, several computer screens display patients' diagnosis and progress, doctors' notes and vital signs such as heart rate and blood pressure. The equipment enables the eICU® doctor to see the patient's medical record including nurse's notes and blood test results. Video conferencing equipment enables two-way conversation between the eICU® doctor and the patient or the family. The eICU® doctor is also able to zoom in on the patient and gauge his or her color and level of consciousness, equipping him with much more information than an average doctor or specialist on call would have. Dedicated hot phones create an instantaneous link between each ICU in the network and the care team in the eICU®. The constant surveillance arms the ICU physician with the patient information needed to make the right decisions and saves lives.

All of these telemedicine applications reduce institutionalized living, allow seniors and people with disabilities to remain active and in the labor force, save individual's time and money, and improve care for many who have not otherwise have access to this level of care. Telemedicine also promises to reduce the cost of care delivery once the initial investment for the infrastructure is paid off.[18]

Key Points

1. Telemedicine is the use of electronic digital technology to provide and support health professionals in their care of patients when distance separates them.
2. Telemedicine depends upon a robust infrastructure that includes the Internet, video, high speed high bandwidth telecommunications, computer-based diagnostics, and various medical devices that enable doctors to do virtual patient examinations and draw adequate conclusions without the elements inherent in the face-to-face meeting.

3. Telemedicine can be delivered via real-time transmission or in an environment where information is received by a consulting physician reviewed and conclusions are forwarded at a later time.

4. One of the growing areas for telemedicine technology is home monitoring where elderly and disabled patients and those with chronic disease use a variety of medical devices in their home to send vital statistics and other information to their doctors or nurses who will contact them if they see an irregularity. This technology saves patients from unnecessary visits to the doctor's office and provides reassurance to those who need constant monitoring.

5. Physicians should understand the needs of these homebound patients and become familiar with the numerous medical devices that offer reliable efficient solutions for monitoring chronic conditions such as diabetes, congestive heart failure, asthma, COPD, and hypertension as well as other serious mechanical conditions and disabilities brought on by neurological diseases, arthritis, etc.

6. Giving every patient access to consults and second opinions is made possible via telemedicine, whether from an urban area or a remote village. However, policy changes regarding reimbursement and licensing of doctors are essential to advancing the use of telemedicine for all underserved populations and individuals who could benefit from these services.

7. Telerehabilitation provides physical therapy, hearing and speech therapy, occupational therapy, mental health services, and hospice services. It enable individuals to remain in their homes or local areas and benefit from services that are simply not available where they live.

8. In an emergency, telemedicine can mean the difference between life and death. The technology is available and the healthcare industry needs to resolve the political and social issues that inhibit trauma telemedicine from working successfully everywhere.

9. The eICU® now enables every patient to have the expertise of an intensive care specialist who monitors and provides appropriate care 24/7.

References and Notes

1. Arizona Telemedicine Newsletter p. 4 "A Life Saved Through Teletrauma Service" www. telemedicine.arizona.edu/updates/page1.htm: also reported at www.federaltelemedicine.com)

2. Telemedicine, TeleHealth, and Health Information Technology, An ATA Issue Paper the American Telemedicine Association May 2006

3. "The Value of Provider-to-Provider TeleHealth Technologies "a study by the Center for Information Technology Leadership p. 69, 2006

4. Centers for Centers for Medicare & Medicaid Services U.S. Department of Health and Human Services www.cms.hhs.gov

5. TeleHealth Connections for Children and Youth, Institute for Child Health Policy, University of Florida, July 2005.

6. Haggerty MC, Stockdale-Woolley R, Nair R. Respi- care: an innovative home care program for the patient with chronic obstructive pulmonary disease. *Chest* 1991;3:607–612.

7. Kornowski R, Zeeli D, Averbuch M, Finkelstein A et al. (Tel Aviv, Israel). Intensive homecare surveillance prevents hospitalization and improved morbidity rates among elderly patients with severe congestive heart failure. *American Heart Journal.* 1995;129(4):762–766.

8. Anecdote published in article in *Harvard Heart Letter*, Volume 15 Number 5, Harvard Medical School, January 2005

9. "Keeping Patients Connected: Technology Helps VA Reduce Hospital Visits," Alice Dembner, Boston Globe, and September 23, 2003.

10. Virtual Medical Worlds Monthly http://www.hoise.com/vmw/06/articles/vmw

11. Based on interview and anecdotal stories from Dr Robert Cox Medical Director at Hays Medical Center in Hays, Kansas

12. Anecdote taken from "Consultations using Telemedicine p. 2 www.teleHealth.hrsa.gov/grants/success.html

13. Anecdotes and facts from interview with Lisa Vetter, Telemedicine Specialist St. Alexius Medical Center

14. http://en.wikipedia.org/wiki/telerehabilitation

15. Based upon interview with Lisa Vetter, Telemedicine Specialist St. Alexius Medical Center

16. http://teleHealth.hrsa.gov/grants/success.htm

17. Kinsella, Audrey"*A Look at New Home Teleinterventions*," Telemedicine, TeleHealth and the Consumer Telehospice: July/August 2004, www.tie.telemed

18. Consultations using Telemedicine http://teleHealth.hrsa.gov/grants/success.htm

Chapter 5
Information Access: Information Overload

The Web is a universal space of information, designed to enable human communication through shared knowledge

Tim Berners-Lee
Director of the World Wide Web Consortium and founder
of the World Wide Web

Healthcare Finds the Internet

A medical doctor who had been in practice over 25 years found out that his son was diagnosed with a rare autoimmune disease about which he knew almost nothing. All of his colleagues in the major medical center where he practiced had little information to offer him. An Internet search provided him and his wife with articles and information that were relevant to their son's disease. It gave them a level of comfort and a lot of information. On the Internet, this doctor identified treatment options that he was able to evaluate. He found discussion groups where he, his wife, and their son could interact with individuals and families facing similar problems. Their son's physician agreed that the information they were unearthing on the Internet was meaningful and helped to map out an overall treatment plan.

The Internet has found its way into healthcare. Built as a tool that scientists could use to facilitate communication with other scientists throughout the world, commercial interests quickly moved in to use the Internet for their business advantage. They put together an infrastructure and they called it the World Wide Web. Soon people everywhere were engaged – some to find information; some to give information; some to interact, to sell, to play, to shop, to lobby, to entertain and be entertained. Web resources enable people to be more informed, more in touch, and more involved with decisions that affect their life. In a health crisis, individuals turn to the Web for accurate facts and constructive advice that could save their life. However, sifting through the great mass of information on the Web is not easy.

N.B. Finn and W.F. Bria, *Digital Communication in Medical Practice*,
DOI: 10.1007/978-1-84882-355-6_6, © Springer-Verlag London Limited 2009

Information Access Telecare Network of North Dakota

A study by the PEW Internet and American Life Project, an independent research group that explores the social impact of the Internet, revealed that on a typical day 75% of American adults log onto the Internet to use email, get news, access government sites, check out health and medical information, participate in auctions, book travel reservations, research their genealogy, gamble, seek out romantic partners, and engage in countless other activities. PEW Internet Project estimates that 80% of Internet users in America or approximately 113 million Americans search the Internet for health information. PEW also found that women are more likely than men to look online for information on most health topics, especially about specific diseases, alternative treatments, diet, nutrition, vitamins, or nutritional supplements. They reported that in a typical Internet health-related search, most individuals spent about 30 minutes and visit two or three sites. Only one in four check the source and date of health information. The research found that the search engines often return dated information.[1]

In another survey, among more than 4,300 US consumers, interviewed by the RAND Corporation for Blue Cross and Blue Shield Association (BCBSA), more than 60% reported searching the Internet for information to help them make healthcare treatment decisions. One-third said the information they found affected their treatment choices or their choice of a healthcare facility. Fifty-two percent said they wanted to make final treatment decisions for themselves or a family member; 38% said they wanted to make the decision together with their physicians.[2]

The American Medical Association reports that on any given day, there are more people online seeking medical advice than actually visit health professionals. It is obvious that consumers, as patients, are actively seeking information about their healthcare options. Among the things Internet users like about being online for healthcare purposes are:

1. The ability to search for health information any time of the day or night.
2. The ability to research a diagnosis or prescription.
3. The ability to prepare for surgery or to find out how to best recover.
4. The readily available tips from caregivers and other patients about specific symptoms, diseases, or problems.
5. The emotional support, stories, good and bad in all sorts of situations.
6. The 24/7-communication channel to keep family and friends informed about the condition of a loved one.

Who Would Benefit Most from Online Access to Health Information?

Figure 5.1 shows results of a survey conducted by the Healthcare Information and Management Systems Society (HIMSS) in December 2007. Nearly half of 187

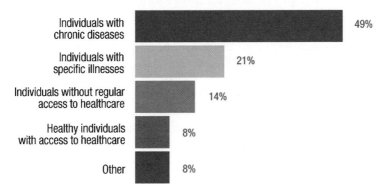

Figure 5.1 Who would benefit the most from online access to health information? © Health information management systems society (HIMSS)

health IT professionals reported that individuals with chronic diseases would be the population that could benefit the most from online access to health information. Twenty-one percent of respondents said individuals with specific illnesses would benefit the most from online access to health information. Nearly half of respondents said the biggest benefit to consumers from expanding the availability of online health care information would be improved care quality. Thirty-five percent of respondents said the greatest benefit would be increased efficiency with administrative quality, while 9% said reduced health care costs.

Information Overload

When Esther and her husband Don had trouble conceiving a baby, they turned to the Internet where they found great comfort in articles that finally explained in lay terms some of the issues that the doctors had been discussing with them. They also found great solace in joining Web groups, checking message boards, and reading posts by other women suffering from infertility who had similar problems to Esther. They were able to download articles they found on the Web and share them together. They found a web community with whom they could discuss these issues. They gained confidence about their treatment choices because they had the information they needed to make sound medical decisions. When they visited their physician, they brought this information into the conversation and asked questions based on what they had learned on the Web.

For years health information was the exclusive province of the healthcare professional. Now it is available everywhere and to everyone. Medical columns in local newspapers and media reports on radio and television appear with increasing frequency; cable television stations air medical programs about operations and procedures with specific graphic details, and offer panel discussions and interviews on a variety of health-related issues; magazines feature in depth reports on health and the consumer is bombarded daily with advertisements of the newly released drugs that promise to cure everything from acne to heart disease. The Internet, with its vast information resources, is where most individuals turn to for health information. This information access has changed the dynamic of health information dissemination. The information patients find on the Internet helps them gain a broader understanding of the health issues they are facing and connects them with a community of other individuals who may be dealing with similar problems. On the one hand, information access is a good thing because it insures a more informed, more healthcare literate patient who is empowered with the intelligence to participate more fully in taking care of themselves and their family. On the other hand, the sheer amount of health-related information present on the Internet and in the media results in information overload. With so much information coming at consumers, it is often difficult for even the most intelligent to filter out what is credible, reliable, and sound information and what is hype.

With this information overload, the twenty-first century healthcare professional has a new task – that of helping patients filter good information in cyberspace from bad information. Every day patients come to their physicians with questions that arise from their health searches on the Internet. As a result physicians need to become familiar with the best sources of health information. Table 5.1 presents guidelines for healthcare professionals who need to assist their patients in finding the right health information resources.

In September 2006, Forrester Research Inc. conducted an online survey of 5,007 US individuals. Among the findings was the fact that consumer access to healthcare information has been increasingly moving online and that consumers report that they are intimidated by the amount of online content available to them and that they do not trust what they see (see Figure 5.2). These same users report that in addition to their online search, they rely on information from their physicians and other healthcare professionals or from family and friends to make

Table 5.1 Criteria for Evaluating Web Sites

1.	Does the Web site state its mission and is it clearly defined as an information resource for healthcare that does not promote products and services?
2.	Does the Web site include site maps and search options for easy navigation?
3.	Is there an indication about when and how often information is updated so it is current?
4.	Does the Web site focus on content that meets a specific need?
5.	Does the Web site link to other information resources that are valuable for the patient?
6.	Does the site include chat rooms and message boards that enable patients to share information?

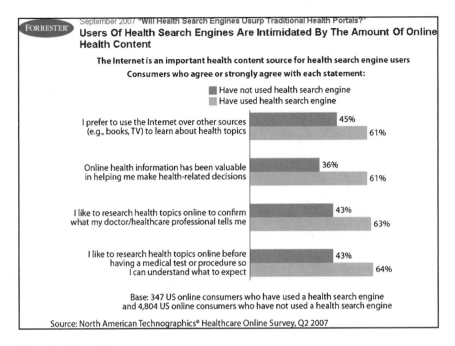

© Forrester Research

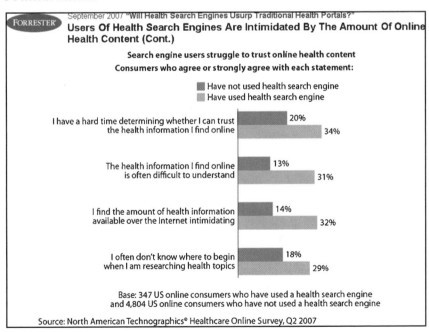

Figure 5.2 Users of health search engines are intimidated by amount of online health content
© Forrester Research

healthcare decisions. The majority of these online healthcare researchers determine content credibility by its affiliation with a well-known research physician or their doctor's endorsement.

Resources for Physicians and Patients

There are many search engines for finding health information. Most of them include similar content: basic information on medications, diseases and conditions, and guidelines on general health issues. The criteria for determining their usefulness is based on how well they organize information and whether or not they include product advertising that would make their information suspect.

http://www.mlanet.org/resources/medspeak/topten.html – This is a site that lists the top ten most useful Web sites according to the Medical Library Association (MLA). These sites were evaluated on the basis of: credibility, sponsorship/authorship, content, audience, currency, disclosure, purpose, links, design, interactivity, and disclaimers by the *Consumer and Patient Health Information Section* of the MLA. They include the following:

http://www.cancer.gov
http://www.cdc.gov
http://www.familydoctor.org
http://healthfinder®.com
http://www.hivinsite.com
http://www.kidshealth®.com
http://www.mayoclinic.com
http://www.medlineplus.com
http://www.medem.com
http://www.noahhealth.org

Each of these sites is covered in depth below, indicated by an asterisk (*)

http://www.uptodate.com

UpToDate is an evidence based, peer reviewed online clinical information resource available to physicians via the Web, desktop, and PDA. *UpToDate* is composed of a synthesis of the literature, the latest evidence, and specific recommendations for patient care, including newly prescribed drugs and newly diagnosed diseases. The *UptoDate* database provides comprehensive coverage on more than 7,000 topics and adding more all the time (more than 75,000 pages of text). These topic reviews are written by several thousand healthcare professionals who are constantly seeking feedback from other user physicians. *UpToDate* is a subscription-based service that accepts no commercial backing or sponsorship content; therefore, recommendations remain free of commercial bias. A patient version is also available.

http://www.healthfinder.com*

Healthfinder® is a "gateway" Web site that links to a broad range of consumer health and human service information resources produced by the Federal Government and its many partner organizations. Healthfinder® was developed by the Department of Health and Human Services and allows the patient to submit Web searches for medical, pharmaceutical, or healthcare information and receive targeted useful health information free of charge. This gateway Web site links to selected online publications, clearinghouses, databases, and over 1,500 Web sites and provides information on every conceivable health topic.

http://www.google.com/Top/Health/

The content of the Google directory based on the Open Directory Project also known as the DMOZ (directory.mozilla.org,) is a multilingual open content directory of World Wide Web links that are constructed and maintained by a community of volunteer editors. The open directory project uses a hierarchical ontology scheme for organizing site listings. The health information search engine includes Harvard Medical School's consumer health information and journal databases and a complete spectrum of health topics for individuals of all ages. Subjects covered include: men and women's' health, health conditions and diseases, health research, informatics, general consumer health concerns such as weight loss and travel health, nutrition, insurance, fitness, cosmetic surgery, medications, and many more. There are also directories of health organizations and links to chats and discussions on health.

http://health.yahoo.com

This Web site is a compendium of everyday health and wellness topics for the consumer including diseases, conditions, fitness, nutrition and articles, and advice on health issues written at a level that patients will understand.

http://www.noahhealth.org*

This site is sponsored by a New York based group of health and science libraries. It is written in both English and Spanish languages and provides 4,000 health/science information links on every topic.

*http://www.medlineplus.gov**

This portal site sponsored by Federal Government branches including the National Library of Medicine and the National Institutes of Health are based upon reliable medically approved information, and addresses topics related to conditions, diseases, and wellness. Over 3,000 doctors, nurse practitioners, and editors contribute content for Medline plus, which is available in both English and Spanish versions. It includes photo illustrations, an extensive drug database and over 4,000 articles about disease, tests, symptoms, as well as a medical encyclopedia and a database of doctors, dentists, and hospitals and clinics. The Medline plus online directory of drugs also includes a database on herbal supplements. The entire site is a great resource for the healthcare professional; however, portions of this site could be too technical for the average consumer.

*http://www.cdc.gov**

This Web site was developed by the Center for Disease Control (CDC) to provide all of the stakeholders in healthcare with information on public health issues. One of the mandates for the CDC is to maintain communications with state and local government agencies, Federal government partners, and the general public. The Web site is the major communication channel to accomplish this and includes: travel alerts related to vaccine requirements, food and beverage precautions, swimming precautions, insect precautions, and disease outbreaks. The CDC Web site also includes podcasts, publications, and discrete sections of information specifically targeted to consumers, healthcare professionals, educators, public health officials, policymakers, researchers, and businesses.

*http://www.familydoctor.org**

This site from the American Academy of Family Physicians takes the patient to links on conditions from A to Z, and includes a patient guide to choosing a family doctor, and a unique set of resources about over the counter solutions to health conditions. It also covers insurance questions, issues of concern regarding Medicare Part D, and other public policy issues of importance to patients. There is a link titled advocacy that enables individuals to send messages to Congress on healthcare issues of concern.

*http://www.medem.org**

This site is covered extensively in Chap. 3 in the section on the eVisit because it is a place where patients and doctors can come together to engage in interactive communication to help patients better manage their health. Medem was founded by the American Medical Association and several national medical specialty societies to develop and provide secure, online communications services for use by physicians and other health-care providers, including hospitals, and health systems, The site includes the option for patients to create an electronic personal health record that is able to accept and transmit information from a patient or physician to an EHR, health plan, pharmacy, and other systems. The site also includes specific patient education programs.

http://www.yourdiseaserisk.com

This site provides a source for information on disease, prevention, and risk for five diseases: cancer, diabetes, heart attack, stroke, and osteoporosis. It includes an interactive tool that measures an individual's risk of these diseases by asking a set of questions and using its intelligence to come up with the risk possibility. The site also provides personalized tips for prevention.

http://www.kidshealth®.com*

This Web site is sponsored and maintained by the Nemours Foundation that sup-ports many health facilities and offers high impact educational programs that affect the health of children. The site's content is divided into three separate sections: *Kids, Teens,* and *Parents* and is written in English and Spanish. A variety of subjects from infections to mental health, from food allergies to managing asthma; from teaching kids about how the body works to helping them understand about drug abuse are addressed. The information posted on this Web site is reviewed by physi-cians on a regular basis.

http://www.physicianreports.com/index

At this site individuals can search by name, state, city to find a doctor, hospital, or nursing home in a particular location in the United States. Thus is particularly use-ful for a patient who is relocating or who lives in more than one location and needs assistance in finding healthcare resources.

http://www.webmd.com

WebMD is probably the most popular health Web site among general consumers and includes timely and relevant news, information and educational materials, video clips, message boards, and healthcare blogs, all of which engage the consumer. Patients can also create a personal health record at WebMD and search for a doctor or hospital. There are many worthwhile tools on the WebMD site that make finding health information both fun and educational, including information on weight and diet, a BMI calculator, advice on dental issues, skin and beauty tips, videos, a symptom checker and more.

Institutional Web Sites

A reliable source of information for patients of a specific hospital or institution are Web sites of that organization and many of them offer not only information that help the patient navigate the system but also general information on health issues as well. These provide a good starting point but may lack the depth of information on the wide range of conditions, diseases, health issues and helpful guidelines and suggestions that patients can find on other sites.

http://www.mayoclinic.com* – The rare exception is the Web site of the Mayo Clinic. The content of this site is credible, reliable, and can compete with any of the health information resources available in cyberspace. In addition to including the standard information about various diseases and drug listings the site includes health tools to monitor disease, discussion options including the ability to chat with a specialist, links to the latest health news, information, blogs, and even a first aid guide.

Professional Organizations

For patients who have a specific health problem, the best sources of information and interactive discussion groups are the sites sponsored by the associations that support those diseases. Some examples include: American Cancer Foundation, http://www.cancer.org, Leukemia & Lymphoma Society http://www.leukemia.org, American Heart Association and American Stroke Association, http://www.americanheart.org, Multiple Sclerosis, http://www.mspathways.com Asthma and Allergies Foundation of America http://www.aafa.org

Online Resources for Cancer

http://www.cancer.gov* – The National Cancer Institute (NCI) was among the first Federal agency to recognize the potential of the Internet for disseminating health-related information. The NCI site is "user driven" and offers cancer patients stakeholder meetings, focus groups, standard and customized online user surveys, usability testing. The site includes information on every type of cancer and discusses new treatments, and clinical trials of new drugs. Cancer patients increasingly turn to the Web in large numbers, seeking to be informed decision makers in their own care. NCI has responded by organizing the CancerNet Web site by audience type with entry points for patients, health professionals, and researchers.

http://www.cancer.org – Cancer patients use Internet resources for general information about the disease as well as for pointers on how to secure a second opinion and how to interpret issues presented by health providers. For patients with rare forms of cancer, the Internet often is the only way to get support and practical advice. This site includes the hard to find information on the financial impact of cancer, and work-related consequences and a comprehensive description of how medical insurance, financial assistance, and cancer intersect. This Web site lists organizations offering financial assistance and provides guidelines for those patients, who need to become familiar with insurance coverage, submit insurance claims, and keep records.

http://www.cancercare.org is another resource for a list of programs offering financial assistance for cancer patients.

Online Resources for Cardiac and Lung Disease

http://www.nhlbi.nih.gov – The National Heart, Lung, and Blood Institute is a good starting place for those who have heart and lung problems. This site offers copious amounts of information on heart attacks, high blood pressure, obesity, cholesterol, asthma, emphysema, lung cancer, and other issues related to health and lung illness. Health assessment tools are also available to help patients assume a more interactive role in learning about specific related issues.

http://www.americanheart.org is also a site with good credible information on cardiac issues.

Online Resources for Diabetes and Kidney Disease

Studies have shown that online programs do work. In one case, patients who participated in an online diabetes education group lowered their blood glucose levels more than they had with other types of controls. Another site for diabetics offered individuals who scuba dive information on to how to cope with their disease 50 feet (15.2 meters) below the water's surface.[3]

http://www.cdc.gov/diabetes (part of the CDC site described above) and **http://www.americandisbetesassociation.org**

These two credible information resources provide patients with educational material that they need to know about diabetes. **http://www.cdc.gov/diabetes** reviews symptoms, types of diabetes, risk factors, treatment options, prevention, and advice. **http://www.americandisbetesassociation.org** provides information on nutrition and weight loss programs, prevention, community education programs, research efforts and more. There are hundreds of other diabetes Web sites some that are reliable and some that offer programs, and products that may not be medically approved. Physicians should caution their patients about using these sites as resources.

Online Resources for HIV

http://www.hivinsite.com* – This is a gateway site, providing information on treatment and prevention, sponsored by the University of California San Francisco School of Medicine and is in the Medical Library Association top ten. It includes links to journal articles and lots of academic-based information and research about HIV.

http://www.thebody.com – Body Health Resources Corporation launched this Web site, *the body.com* for HIV positive individuals 10 years before drugs were available to prolong the lives of so many people dying of AIDS, when there was virtually little information available. Over 500,000 unique visitors come to *thebody. com* every month – three quarters from the US and the rest from around the world. A third of these visitors are people diagnosed with HIV; others are care givers/partners of HIV positive individuals and medical professionals. Over 16,000 doctors and nurses provide updates to the body.com. Moderated and unmoderated message boards and a variety of educational forums and materials are also available.

The Internet is full of weight loss advice and services to address the massive problem of weight control. For many adults, there are reasons why online diet programs are appealing. They are convenient and can be accessed 24/7. They offer patients anonymity and some of these sites include useful tools that allow patients to track their progress, which hopefully increases their' motivation to stick with a program. The three Web sites listed offer resources that are credible, reliable, and do not sell products. They provide a good starting point for the patient who is seeking weight loss advice and tools via the Internet.

http://www.eatright.org/public/
http://www.obesity.org
http://www.mayoclinic.com

Online Resources for Ordering Drugs

PEW research studies identified that nearly one half of American adults or about 91 million people take prescription drugs on a regular basis and one in four Americans have looked online for drug information. PEW found that only a fraction of Americans has ever bought prescription drugs online.[4]

As the cost of drugs continues to rise, and access to new drugs is limited and delayed by both patients' health insurers and by the US Food and Drug Administration (FDA) clinical trial and approval process, more and more individuals are going online to try to find cost effective remedies that may not always be what their physician would recommend. Patients need to be educated to identify safe and responsible Web resources. They need to be taught to avoid those Web sites that sell products that could endanger their health. Physicians have a responsibility to remind their patients that reputable Web sites require that prescriptions are written by a patient's health provider and adhere to regulations enforced by government agencies such as state pharmaceutical boards and the US Food and Drug Administration (FDA). It is important for physicians to warn their patients that prescription drugs can be purchased at sites located in countries where there are few if any laws or enforced policies regarding the content of those advertised drugs. These compounds may be compromised in dosage as well as formula.

Safe sites will have an insignia on the site that reflects the drug industry's self-regulation mechanisms such as the Verified Internet Pharmacy Practice Site "VIPPS" run by the National Association of Boards of Pharmacy. The FDA publishes a warning for consumers buying medical products online at **http://www.fda. gov/oc/buyonline/default.ht.** The site includes a list of all drugs. By clicking on an individual drug the site will take the visitor to a page that provides a complete overview of the drug and its adverse effects.

http://www.drugs.com – This is a comprehensive site for patients who want to research medications and their side effects and check drug interactions

http://www.rxlist.com – This spin off of WebMD provides a drug index as well as new information about drugs. However, patients are cautioned that there is advertising on the site.

http://www.druginfonet.com

This Web site advertises itself as a free resource for a more informed consumer, and it lives up to its promise. Frequently asked questions, drug information, health information, a full database of information about drug manufacturers (pharmaceutical companies), health news stories, and much more makes this a viable information resource for patients. It is certified by HON code standard for trustworthy health information and Trustee certified privacy standards. The site does advertise products and links to advertised products for specific conditions

The list of Web sites is by no means a complete list of all of the resources on the Web as there are thousands to choose from and many are excellent. By following the specific guidelines listed below, physicians can advise their patients to help them navigate the Web with confidence that the information they find will be accurate and useful.

Specific guidelines for Web information include:

1. **Choose trustworthy sites of established healthcare organizations.**

The ". *gov*"sites sponsored by Federal, state, or local government or reputable govt. agencies, e.g. HHS, CDC, and NIH are credible and will not advertise products. They can be held to the test for accuracy, reliability, and impartiality.

The Web sites of medical publications: *New England Journal of Medicine, Journal of the American Pediatrics Society. where* information is supplied by doctors and researchers and is peer reviewed. These are sites specifically for a physician audience and are typically beyond the grasp of the average patient.

Specific disease searches are most efficient at the Web sites of the not-for-profit societies: the American Cancer Society, the Leukemia Society, and The Brain Tumor Society. They have a vested interested in helping physicians and patients find information of value.

2. Look for Seals of Approval – there are three worth noting:

Health-On-The-Net Foundation (HON) is a nongovernmental nonprofit foundation, supported by the United Nations Economic and Social Council and designed to guide consumers to reliable, credible health, and medical information on the Internet.

Hi-Ethics, Inc., or Health Internet Ethics, unites the most widely used health Internet sites supporting high ethical standards. Member companies are committed to earning the trust and confidence of consumers who choose to use Internet health services for improving their health and healthcare.

Internet Healthcare Coalition (IHCC), the IHCC is an independent and non-industry aligned group. Dedicated to educating healthcare consumers, professionals, educators, marketers, and both healthcare and mainstream media, as well as public policymakers on the full range of uses of the Internet – current and potential – to deliver high-quality healthcare information and services.

3. Ask the following questions when looking for the appropriate Web site:

Who developed this site? Is the organization clearly identified? Are the credentials of the authors of papers listed?

Does the page show when it was last updated? Are the links to other resources active?

Is contact information provided so that you can email call or write the Web sponsor?

What is the purpose of the information?

Can the information be verified in other sources?

4. Beware of Web sites that make promises and use medical jargon

Physicians must advise patients to be wary of any Web site that offers remedies that result in fast weight loss, instant hair replacement, miracle cures, nutritional supplements, great healing remedies. They also have an obligation to warn patients to be especially careful of sites that try to sell products, vitamins, and health services.[5]

Key Points

1. The twenty-first century eHealth Professional is forced to recognize that patients are seeking health information on the Web and looking to their physicians for guidance about how to use the Web effectively.

2. The best way to assist patients is to supply them with an information sheet that lists credible Web sites that the physician or a member of the staff has reviewed for accuracy, timeliness, and authenticity.
3. For every medical situation, there is too much information; some of it is good information, a lot of it bad information. The healthcare professional should not assume that patients are able to distinguish among good and the bad.
4. The Web can be most beneficial to patients with chronic diseases who can use the information resources on the Web to stay abreast of the latest developments with their condition, connect with others who have the same condition, and find Web tools that can help them better monitor their condition.
5. Physicians need to warn their patients to be wary of general search engine results that can populate a page with links to information that is out of date, unreliable, and inaccurate.
6. Government and healthcare institutional Web sites are generally accurate as are those of health insurers, and those sponsored by not-for-profit health organizations and professional associations and therefore offer the best resources.

References and Notes

1. Pew Internet & American Life Project, October 24 – December 2, 2007 Tracking Survey. N = 2,054 adults, 18 and older. Margin of error is ± 2% for results based on the full sample and ± 3% for results based on internet users.
2. Journal of the American Medical Informatics Association Volume 11 Number 6, Nov/Dec, 2004. www.consumeraffairs.com/news/2005/rand_health_info.html
3. McKay HG King D, Eakin EG Seeley JR Glasgow RE. The diabetes network Internet base activity intervention: a randomized pilot study. *Diabetes Care* 2001;24(8):1328-1334
4. Prescription Drugs Online by Susannah Fox, Pew Internet and American Life Project, October 2004
5. Evaluating Health Web Sites, Jana Liebermann Consumer Health Coordinator NNLM Southeastern Atlantic Region

Chapter 6
Keeping Health Information Away from Prying Eyes

William E. Alberts was a minister with the Southern New England Conference of the United Methodist Church. He engaged the services of Donald T. Devine for the provision of psychiatric services. Alberts assumed that implicit in their relationship was the understanding that Dr. Devine would keep confidential all information, observations, and opinions relating to the diagnosis, condition, behavior, and treatment of Alberts. However, in April 1973, Dr. Devine disclosed to Resident Bishop Edward G. Carroll of the Boston Area of the United Methodist Church and John E. Barclay, President of the United Methodist Conference, information about Albert's diagnosis, condition, behavior, and treatment. That information was then passed along to members of various boards, committees, and subcommittees of the United Methodist Church Conference. Additionally, Bishop Carroll informed the news media that Alberts was "mentally ill and therefore was not to be re-appointed as a minister."

These actions caused considerable loss of earning capacity and other financial losses to Minister Alberts, in addition to damaging his reputation and causing great mental anguish requiring further medical treatment. He brought legal action against Dr. Donald Devine, Bishop Carroll, and John Barclay. The case went to the Massachusetts Supreme Judicial Court.

The Court held that the confidentiality between a doctor and his patient was inviolate, stating: "exception to the rule of confidentiality when aspects of an employee's health could affect an employee's ability to effectively perform job duties is not so broad as to permit a physician to disclose to a patient's employer whether information might bear on the employee's ability to perform job duties."[1]

In several other cases, the courts have also imposed on physicians a duty of confidentiality, maintaining that public policy favors the protection of a patient's right to confidentiality. The New Jersey Supreme Court reinforced this principle in Bratt v. International Business Machine Corporation stating:

> *"A patient should be entitled to freely disclose his symptoms and condition to his doctor in order to receive proper treatment without fear that those facts may become public property. Only thus can the purpose of the relationship be fulfilled."[2]*

N.B. Finn and W.F. Bria, *Digital Communication in Medical Practice,*
DOI: 10.1007/978-1-84882-355-6_7, © Springer-Verlag London Limited 2009

Medical Information is no Longer Private

Privacy is defined as excluded or isolated from view or contact with others. In the twenty-first century medical practice, where numerous tests and procedures have become routine and referral to specialists by a primary care doctor is standard practice, information about patients' passes through the hands of faceless workers and institutions such as labs, hospitals, payers, and others. Typically, an individual's medical record contains a description of symptoms, medical history, examination and test results, diagnoses, treatment, medications, payment data, benefits coordination, health plan eligibility, referral certification, and authorization. The individual's social security number, birth date, and other relevant conditions may also be noted in that record. Third party reimbursement, managed care, email communications, health information exchange, electronic medical and personal health records, and other ehealth initiatives raise questions about how easily that health information can be penetrated and tampered with by unauthorized individuals. Paper files do not fare any better. When a patient goes to the emergency room of a community hospital that does not have an electronic health record, a paper chart is created that goes with the patient wherever he or she is transported. This entire record could be viewed by as many as 100 healthcare workers including doctors-in-training, attending physicians, nurses and technicians in all of the labs that the patient visits. On the general medical ward, the record is available to nurses, nursing assistants, residents, attending physicians, and specialists who come to the floor to check on the patient. It is also available to personnel who transport the individual to therapists, labs, and social workers. Paper files of outpatients that live on desks and in drawers in a physician's office can also be accessed if someone deliberately wants to get to them.

Confidentiality, which has always been the basis of a doctor-patient relationship and is defined as *"ensuring that information is accessible only to those authorized to have access,"* is inherent in the way that medical institutions and payers handle patient information. In some instances, there are overriding legitimate reasons why health information must be shared: to insure that the patient will receive necessary treatment or to insure that the society is properly protected. There have been instances where the courts have held that doctors have an obligation to pass on information to protect nonpatients, for example, where the doctor must warn police of a mentally unstable patient who has threatened a specific person with violence. The current health reimbursement system that involves third parties requires that doctor's transmit medical information to payers as a condition of coverage and as a safeguard against fraud and overpayment. Blood work and other tests are often sent to laboratories for analysis where the patient's health information is viewed and analyzed by numerous individuals. What is critical to the process is to maintain confidentiality and ensure that personal information does not enter the public domain. The resolution of how individuals' rights are handled and weighed against the legitimate need for provider and payer information concerning coverage and treatment, as well as oversight of these relationships is still evolving. At the Federal level, there is the Health Insurance Portability and Accountability Act (HIPAA) (discussed later in this chapter), which is a first step in trying to impose a coherent and principled framework for analyzing these issues.

Privacy Issues Concern Physicians and Patients

Physicians have been slow to adopt electronic health records and privacy concerns have been among their top concerns. Their patients also take the threat to privacy of health information very seriously. In a survey conducted in 2005 by Princeton Survey Research Associates for the California HealthCare Foundation, respondents viewed computerization of medical information as the most serious threat to privacy. Although most patients trust their doctors to keep their information private, the survey revealed that most Americans distrust private health insurance plans and government health programs when it comes to keeping personal medical information private and confidential. Over 50% of respondents said that they worry about computer hackers breaking into a system that contains their medical records. That same group indicated that they trust doctors, hospitals, and other health professionals to keep personal information confidential all or most of the time. Nearly 10% of the respondents of this study had experienced an improper disclosure that resulted in personal embarrassment or harm.[3]

Even the government, the entity that physicians and patients would assume to be the overseer and protector of the publics' health information, has violated that trust. There have been several instances where attorneys for the United States Justice Department attempted to thwart privacy protections and obtain medical records. These actions were in relation to the records held by Planned Parenthood clinics, and related to women who had or were planning abortions. The records sought were paper and the Justice Department argued that the names could have been removed to protect the identification of the individuals involved. But had they been electronic, the names could not have been removed and the question remains, whether or not an electronic health record could have made it easier for the government to pry. The Department justified their actions and contended that Federal law does not recognize a physician-patient privilege in these instances. In most states, the Courts have fortunately disagreed, blocking the Department's demand for access to these records.[4]

Electronic health records are generally accessed using a password protected system. Individuals with a need to see the record are typically granted access to only selective parts of the record instead of full access to the whole chart. Audit trails closely monitor who has viewed the record. Even with these protections the same electronic information that sits behind firewalls and is encrypted has been subject to tampering by computer savvy individuals who know how to hack into databases to get what they want, and even by curiosity seekers who may have access to a record but do not have a need-to-know the information.

Between 2005 and 2006, the personal information of more than one in four Americans – 85 million people – was compromised. One of the most publicized and outrageous incident's was the theft of a single Veterans' Administration laptop with the Social Security numbers and medical information of 26.5 million people that took place in the spring of 2006. An employee of the VA took the data home without authorization. The information was returned without damage to the security of the individuals' medical information on that laptop. This violation of confidentiality is exactly the fear expressed by healthcare professionals who have not moved their files from paper to digital format or who have done so reluctantly.

Health information is not just in the hands of the doctor. Most health plans have vast information about their individual subscribers, accumulated from payment and approval records that include doctors' fees, lab fees, charges for procedures, in-hospital stays, surgeries, and pharmaceutical charges. Legally, covered entities (health plans including employer sponsored health plans, Medicare and Medicaid) may use and disclose personal health information for treatment, payment, and operations of the covered entities. They may also disclose personal health information to third parties that perform services for them, such as a disease management, utilization review, or quality assurance organizations, without individual authorization, as long as there is a HIPAA-required business associate agreement in place. There are specific rules regarding what information an employer may obtain from an employer-sponsored group health plan. They are generally limited to enrollment payment and summary health information to administer the plan.

Protecting Data with a Secure Network

Security of computer networks is a first line of defense in protecting information. This security is based on firewalls and authentication techniques that build in controls to confirm: (1) the identity of the person requesting access to information; (2) uniform methods to authorize and control access; (3) aggressive software management, and (4) regular monitoring to check for vulnerability. Firewalls are built from hardware, software, and network equipment to permit certain access and deny other traffic. They range from the simple to the complex, and act as automated security guards or censors, scanning traffic, from and to the Internet, and permitting only that which meets specified criteria. No matter how complex a firewall is, there are ways to break through it.

A problem unique to healthcare organizations is that they traditionally distribute confidential information across many media. Patient medical records that incorporate waivers, charts, audio files, photographs, notes and other confidential information types are stored on network drives. There are also handheld devices, local hard drives, picture archiving and communication systems (PACS), X-ray equipment and, of course, scanned physical records that send and receive information through the network. Although central files exist, the lack of access, control, and detailed audit trails on these diverse devices make this information vulnerable.

The three major concerns regarding network security are the following:

Malware

Viruses, Trojan horses, worms, spyware, and other forms of malicious software pose a major threat to the security of a network. Anti-virus and anti-spyware products help, but they only treat the symptoms of infection instead of the cause. By reinforcing computers with the appropriate security configurations, organizations can eliminate the vast majority of system vulnerabilities that malware exploits.

Automatic Log-off

Workers in healthcare settings often leave their computer workstations without logging off. This poses a security risk, to health information, particularly when the workstation is in an area accessible to unauthorized people. Adding an automatic log-off feature to every computer in a system can solve this problem. The HIPAA Security Rule states that covered entities must implement electronic procedures that terminate an electronic session after a predetermined period of inactivity.

Theft of Removable Media

The proliferation of USB devices such as thumb drives, flash drives, and MP3 players create a situation where data can be downloaded to these tiny devices and stolen with the click of a mouse. Patient files, folders, and personal information residing on the computers at HMOs, hospitals, and other healthcare organizations are at risk for this type of invasion.

All of these concerns can be addressed with appropriate safeguards and oversight by the IT team. Training of the individuals involved in providing and using healthcare IT systems is essential and cannot be emphasized enough. This training should include discussions with healthcare workers in every facet of a healthcare organization, about how to protect patient information and use of computers and other information storage devices. Healthcare organizations must implement more stringent controls over who has access to computer equipment that houses medical records and how much information can be released from these systems to comply with privacy regulations.

US Federal Regulations Regarding Privacy (HIPAA)

The Congress of the United States, in 1996, enacted the Health Insurance Portability and Accountability Act (HIPAA). HIPAA has two parts. Title I of HIPAA protects health insurance coverage for workers and their families when they change or lose their job. Title II of HIPAA, The Administration Simplification (AS) provisions require the establishment of national standards for electronic health care transactions and national identifiers for providers, health insurance plans, and employers. These provisions have been expanded to apply to paper information as well. The AS provisions also address the security and privacy of health data, particularly health data that exists in digital format and sets civil and criminal penalties for offenses relating to healthcare information and privacy violations. As the number of consumers connecting with physicians online has increased incrementally each year since the beginning of the twenty-first century (Figure 6.1), HIPAA has become more important as a safeguard for the individual's health information. These rules apply to covered entities: insurers and health plans including Medicare, Tricare, state Medicaid plans, commercial health plans, and employers sponsored group health plans; healthcare clearinghouses such as billing services; community health information systems and health care providers that transmit personal information electronically in connection with certain enumerated standard transactions, e.g., electronic claims submissions and referral requests.

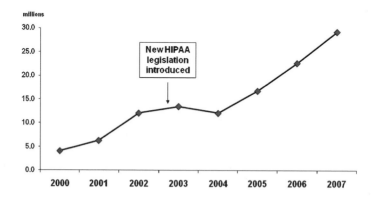

Figure 6.1 The health insurance portability and accountability act of 1996 – HIPAA

The Privacy Rule

In 2003, the Privacy Rule was promulgated to establish a national floor of privacy protections for patients by limiting the ways that health plans, pharmacies, hospitals, and other covered entities can use and disclose to third parties patients' personal medical information. It also includes a provision that enables patients to both access their medical records and control how their personal health information is used and disclosed. Medical records and other individually identifiable health information, whether on paper, in computers or communicated orally, are included in the Privacy Rule protection. A key premise of the Privacy Rule is to assure that individuals' health information is properly protected while allowing the flow of health information needed to provide and promote high quality healthcare that assures the public's health and well being.

The specifics of the Privacy Rule include:

1. Each covered entity with certain exceptions must provide a notice of privacy to its practices. The Privacy Rule requires that the notice contain certain elements. The notice must describe ways in which the covered entity may use and disclose protected health information. The notice must state the covered entities duties to protect privacy, provide a notice of privacy practices, and abide by the terms of the current notice. The notice must describe individuals' rights including the right to complain to the HHS and to the covered entity if they believe their privacy rights have been violated. The notice must include a point of contact for further information and for making complaints to the covered entity.[5]

2. Patient Access to Medical Records: Upon request patients must be given control over how their personal health information is used and disclosed. They have the right to see their medical information, to copy, and supplement but not to change their medical records. They have the authority to refuse to have certain individuals or organization see their records.

3. Appropriate Safeguards: HIPAA states emphatically that healthcare providers, health plans and information clearing houses that collect, share, and store health information must have appropriate technical and administrative safeguards in place to protect that information. Alternative means of communication such as email may be used only with appropriate safeguards.

4. Limits on use of personal medical information: The Privacy Rule sets limits on how health plans and providers may use individually identifiable health information. On the one hand, to promote the best quality care for patients, the rule does not restrict the ability of doctors, nurses, and other providers to share information needed to treat their patients. On the other hand, personal health information generally may not be disclosed to a patient's employer without written consent, nor may it be used for purposes not related to health care. Information may be shared with a family member or other designated close friend or relative, with the patient's consent. That individual may act on behalf of the patient to pick up prescriptions, medical supplies, and provide other needed health assistance.

Covered entities may use or share only the minimum amount of protected information needed for a particular purpose. Given these limitations set forth by the Privacy Rule, physicians should make a point of encouraging every patient to provide them with a signed healthcare proxy.

5. Limits on use of health information for marketing purposes: The Privacy Rule sets restrictions so that patients must sign a specific authorization before a covered entity can release their medical information to a life insurer, a bank, a marketing firm, or anyone else not directly involved in their healthcare. Although doctors and other covered entities are permitted to communicate freely with patients about treatment options and other health-related information, including disease-management programs, marketing of patient information is not allowed.

6. Confidential communications: Under the Privacy Rule, patients can request that their doctors, health plans, and other covered entities take reasonable steps to ensure that their communications are confidential. For example, a patient could ask a doctor to call his or her office rather than home, and the doctor's office should comply with that request if it can be reasonably accommodated.

7. Complaints: Doctors must comply with the privacy rules and should check in frequently at the HHS Website for changes in the rule. A patient who has concerns about privacy may file a complaint with their health plan or directly with the United States Department of Health and Human Services Office for Civil Rights (OCR). Information on filing and updates to the Privacy Rule can be found at http://www.hhs.gov/ocr/discrimhowtofile.html.

Under state law there are common law (case law) rights to privacy, medical record statutes, and confidentiality obligations under professional standards and licensing laws. There are also a growing number of states that have enacted identity theft laws that contain similar but not the same mitigation obligations as HIPAA for privacy breaches.[6]

The Specific Benefits of this Federal and State Legislation include:

- Specific boundaries on the use and release of health records.
- Appropriate safeguards that healthcare providers and others must achieve to protect the privacy of health information.
- Civil and criminal penalties that hold violators accountable, including criminal penalties (prison time up to 10 years) and fines up to $250,000 for knowingly misusing individually identifiable health information.
- Parameters when disclosure of some forms of data is determined to be essential to protect public health.
- Rules on disclosure and use of patient information.
- Limitations on the amount of information released.
- Patient rights to examine and obtain copies of their own health records and request corrections.
- Patient empowerment to control certain uses and disclosures of their health information

The European Union on Privacy

US privacy protections are not actually considered to be as robust as privacy laws governing the dissemination of health information in other countries. The European Union for example has taken a very strong position on protecting the individual. The EU's comprehensive privacy legislation, the Directive on Data Protection (the Directive), became effective on October 25, 1998. Article 25 of the EU Directive prohibits any EU country from transferring personal data via the Internet to, or receiving data from, countries deemed to lack "adequate" Internet privacy protection. Although the United States and the European Union share the goal of enhancing privacy protection for their citizens, the United States takes a different approach to privacy that relies on a mix of legislation, regulation, and self regulation. The European Union's rules are specific and inviolate and essentially prohibit member states from processing any personal data concerned with health issues.

The Internet

In twenty-first century healthcare, there is a new privacy dilemma for ehealth professionals and their patients – the increasing use of the Internet for the collection, storage and communication of medical and other personal records. Internet access potentially enables agencies, institutions, and strangers throughout the world to view medical records. Large databases that include these records are stored and can be accessed via the Internet. Some physicians and patients use the World Wide Web and not a secure portal to send and receive messages containing health information. Compounding the problem is the fact that many patients are forced to provide personal health information to gain employment, procure insurance, obtain a credit card, or participate in today's economy. The bureaucratic institutions that control and use that information offer virtually no accountability or rationale in why or how the information will be used.[7]

A Forrester Research study conducted in January 2007 (Figure 6.2) found that consumers are reluctant to use a PHR that is sponsored by a health plan because they fear these sites are not secure enough to prevent malevolent outsiders from accessing and misusing their data and thus violating their privacy.

Email

Judy, 44, a senior analyst at a large financial institution was in line for a promotion when she learned that she had a fairly uncommon type of Breast Cancer. Naturally she was devastated. However, her doctor assured her that with the early diagnosis and proper, swift medical treatment she would have a good chance of full recovery.

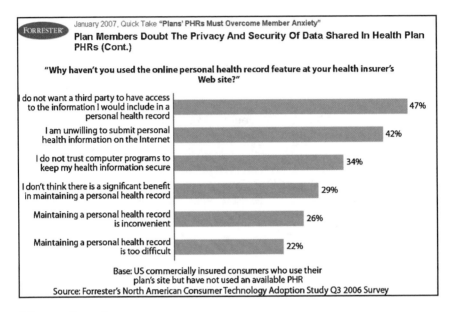

© Forrester Research

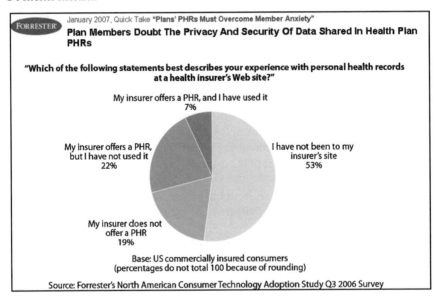

Figure 6.2 Plan members doubt the privacy and security of data shared in health plan PHRS "Why haven't you used the online personal health record feature at your health insurer's Web site?" © Forrester Research

Knowing that Judy was the type of patient that had to learn everything about her diagnosis, the doctor gave her several links to medical Web sites and told her to email him with questions.

Judy returned to her office, anxious, but determined. During her lunch break, she did an extensive Web search to gather as much information as she could about her illness. Once she was satisfied, she formulated her questions and emailed her doctor from the office computer. A week later, Judy had a meeting with the Vice President of her division for her annual performance review. Although she had excellent ratings on every facet of her work, her supervisor hesitated when Judy asked him about the promotion. When pressed, the supervisor explained the company's executive committee was concerned that Judy's illness might prevent her from meeting the demands placed upon her that included long hours and travel. Judy was shocked. She immediately realized that her Web search had been tracked and her email to her doctor read, violating her privacy. Dismayed and angry she brought her concerns to the human resources department. She contended that the company had never issued a policy to its employees warning that Web searches or emails through the company server, conducted on the employee's own time, could be monitored and used against her. She argued that the company had a moral obligation to warn employees if personal communications were going to be viewed by anyone. Caught in a no-win situation, Judy had the choice to ignore the violation to her privacy, keep her job and hopefully her promotion or to contest the company's violation of her privacy by retaining an attorney, issuing an official complaint, or even suing.

Judy's woes are not unique. Most people are aware that the company they work for owns the computer they are using and if they want to maintain the privacy of their data they should not be sending emails to their doctor with private information. However, that does not give the company the right to snoop either. There are numerous examples where there are questionable actions regarding violation of personal privacy by individuals, healthcare organizations, healthcare workers, employers, and media, even by what patients consider a benign organization such as their neighborhood CVS pharmacy.

Most email messages transmitted over the World Wide Web are not encrypted, and thus are subject to interception by unauthorized individuals. HIPAA specifically states that healthcare providers are allowed to use alternative means of communication, such as email as long as they maintain appropriate safeguards that "ensure the confidentiality, integrity, and availability" of any health information transmitted electronically, and "protect against any reasonably anticipated threats" to the security of such information." To meet these requirements, email users can encrypt their messages. Encryption is a process that uses sophisticated software with cryptographic algorithms to garble words. Encryption assumes that the recipient has the correct digital key to unscramble and read the message. Particularly vulnerable to a communication on the Internet are the points where the communication enters or leaves a device on the communications path. Individuals wanting to hack into a message to acquire data, eavesdrop on audio

Table 6.1 Patient Guidelines for Email Communications

1. Never assume that an email will remain confidential.
2. Do not use email for situations where you need a quick response.
3. Do not use email for sensitive issues that you want to keep confidential.
4. Always include your name; **never** include your social security number or telephone number in an email that is not encrypted.
5. If you really want privacy do not use email, call.
6. Keep copies of emails you send to physicians or other healthcare providers.

transmission, or view an entire audio/video care delivery process can do so. When employees send an email through the company server, as Judy did, those emails can also be intercepted and read. All of these factors contribute to many physicians' reluctance to use email communications with their patients unless they have access to a secure portal that enables secure messaging. Table 6.1 provides guidelines that physicians give to patients who insist on email communication:

Questionable Privacy Practices

For purposes of disease management, there are many instances where information on patients is shared with every good intention. The good that accrues from these activities to the patient population can outweigh any threats to privacy, but it is a slippery slope that must be approached with care. In many clinical studies, patients, with permission, allow their data to be used. Generally, there is a real effort to scrub that data so that names and specific identification are not possible; however, there is always the chance that certain information could be traced back to an individual. The Center for Medicare and Medicaid Services (CMS) has amassed databases that gather information to aid plans, physicians, and providers to improve quality; and to help Medicare beneficiaries and other consumers, health plans and other purchasers make informed choices. This "Quality Initiatives Research" is based primarily on information gathered directly from patients. These data are scrubbed so it is not likely that anything could be traced to specific information about individuals but privacy issues loom whenever government collects that type of information, even if it is intended to benefit the public.

Case Study: CVS

CVS implemented a Patient Compliance Program to provide health care information to its pharmacy customers. Using a database prepared from customers' prescription records, a third party company, on CVS's behalf, mailed letters to several of its pharmacy customers. Those customers were not previously informed of, or asked to consent to this program. The mailings concerned drugs and medical conditions and took a variety of forms. Some letters provided information on the risks of certain health conditions; some letters urged customer to switch to a new or alternative prescription medication; one mailing addressed the benefits of taking and refilling prescriptions. Each letter included a box to check if the customer did not want to receive further mailings. Although the letters were written on CVS pharmacy letterhead, the mailings were financed by several drug manufacturers.

Jeffrey Kelley filled his diabetes medicine at CVS. The letter he received talked about the dangers of high cholesterol that is a known risk for diabetes patients. The letter was clearly marked, "sponsored by Merck and Company Inc.," a manufacturer of the anti-cholesterol prescription drug Zocor. Kelley felt that the letter invaded his privacy and, along with other individuals who had received letters, initiated a class action lawsuit against CVS and the pharmaceutical companies who had participated in the program. They argued that CVS and the pharmaceutical companies, for their own financial gain, improperly used confidential medical information provided to CVS by its pharmacy customers, thus violating the privacy rights of those customers.[8]

The court held that the letter did not violate Mr. Kelley's right to privacy. In Massachusetts, an invasion of privacy requires an "unreasonable, substantial, or serious interference" with privacy. In this case, CVS did not disclose Mr. Kelley's name to Merck, and only provided his name, date of birth, and address (all of which is public information). The third party mail house, Elensys did not know why Mr. Kelley had been selected to receive the letter and did not receive any information about his medical or pharmaceutical history. The court reasoned that there is nothing improper about a pharmacy reviewing its prescription database and providing relevant information to its customers, and that the fact that CVS used a third party to do this was essentially the same as hiring extra clerks to send the information directly from the pharmacy. The court also noted that Mr. Kelley "readily disclosed" his diabetes to friends and associates, which made it "even clearer that the information disclosed by CVS cannot reasonably be deemed a substantial or serious interference with his privacy." The court, however, did find that CVS engaged in an unfair and deceptive act by concealing the fact that it profited from sending the letters.[9]

The Dilemma

Privacy is a difficult issue. On the one hand, as a society we cannot afford to halt progress by refusing to use electronic technology or disallowing data to be electronically stored on databases. On the other hand, the risk that the data could be abused never quite goes away. In 1977, a group of patients and prescribing doctors brought an action challenging the constitutionality of a New York State statute that gives the State the right to maintain a database of patient names, addresses, and ages of people who use the most dangerous legitimate drugs. These data are filed with the New York State Health Department and kept for a five-year period using a system that is supposed to safeguard the security of the information, after which it is destroyed. Public disclosure of the patient's identity is prohibited and access to the files is confined to a limited number of health department and investigatory personnel.

The case regarding the existence of this database and the privacy questions involved was heard by the United States Supreme Court: Whalen v. Roe, 429 US 589 (1977). In a unanimous decision, the Court decreed that the New York program does not, on its face, pose a sufficient threat to establish a constitutional violation. The Court noted that that the State's carefully designed program includes numerous words and safeguards intended to forestall the danger of indiscriminate disclosure.

> "We hold, that neither the immediate nor the threatened impact of the patient identification requirements in the New York State Controlled Substances Act of 1972 on either the reputation or the independence of patients for whom Schedule II drugs are medically indicated, is sufficient to constitute an invasion of any right or liberty protected by the Fourteenth Amendment."[10]

In a perfect world, we would have the efficiency and economies that digital technology brings to information management, collection and storage, and the privacy protections that always insure that the data can not be penetrated or disturbed. However, it is not a perfect world. The digital accumulation of data has moved at a much faster pace than the ability of the same digital technology to protect that data. As the cases discussed show, there are also many gray areas where privacy issues are concerned. Therefore, the best that healthcare organizations, groups, institutions, and society can do is to use all the available protections and surveillance systems available while living with the constant awareness that there are threats to health information data lurking at all times.

Key Points

1. There are many external influences that threaten to erode the confidentiality of patient information including the imposition of third-party reimbursement, managed care, digital technology, and the complexity of providing healthcare to patients in the twenty-first century.
2. Physicians and their patients often have no control over who sees the medical information of the patient, whether it is on paper or in digital format. As an in-patient as many as 100 healthcare professionals could see the record at one time or another during a hospital stay. In the outpatient setting, patient's health information or part of it is seen not only within the physician's office but also by numerous health payers, pharmacists, specialty healthcare providers and others, creating a privacy dilemma that has no solution.
3. The first line of protection for health information is to be sure that patient's health information resides on a secure network with the appropriate firewalls and authentication procedures in place.
4. The Federal Government's concern with privacy issues related to health information led to the passage of the Health Insurance Portability and Accountability Act of 1996 and the Privacy Rule in 2003. These pieces of legislation along with individual state regulations are based on privacy protections inherent in the

United States Constitution and attempt to address digital technology in health information management and dissemination. The European Union has even more stringent requirements concerning privacy.

5. Email use is of particular concern as it relates to privacy of patient health information. Email sent over the public Internet is at greater risk of landing in the wrong hands than email set through a secure messaging system such as a health-care portal.

6. There are many gray areas regarding an individual's privacy of health information as indicated by the Court's view in the CVS case where the Court concluded that a health entity (pharmacy in this case) can use a database of names, addresses, and diagnoses to send marketing materials to those individuals as long as the details of their medical record are not revealed.

7. Health information privacy issues continue to warrant oversight, discussion, and concern and healthcare professionals are at the forefront of that debate.

References and Notes

1. William E. Alberts vs. Donald T. Devine et al. Massachusetts, Supreme Judicial Court Norfolk County, Boston MA, Westlaw 395 Mass.59479 N.E 2d 113
2. Bratt v. International Business Machs. Corp., 467 N.E. 2d 126 at 522-523. quoting Hogue v. Williams 37 NJ 328, 336,181A2d345(1962)
3. National Consumer Health Privacy Project Survey, 2005, California Healthcare Foundation. www.chef.org/topics/view.cfm?itemID=19746
4. *The New York Times*, "When Big Brother Invades the Examining Room," Howard Markel, MD, March 16, 2004
5. The United states Department of Health and Human Services OCR (Office for Civil Rights) Privacy Brief, Summary *of the HIPAA Privacy Rule State Regulations April 2003, 11*
6. The United states Department of Health and Human Services OCR (Office for Civil Rights) Privacy Brief, Summary *of the HIPAA Privacy Rule State Regulations April 2003*, www.hhs. gov/ocr/privacysummary/pdf
7. Solove DJ. *The Digital Person: Technology and Privacy in the Information Age*, New York: New York University Press; 2004:51.
8. Weld and Kelly vs. CVS Pharmacy, Inc., et al: Civil Action No. 98-0897-F, Superior Court Department of the Trial Court, Commonwealth of Massachusetts.
9. FDA Law Blog Hyman Phelps and McNamara P.C. "Mass Court Permits Pharmacy Mailing Program but Requires Disclosure of Profits" October 22, 2006, www.fdalawblog.net
10. http://biotech.law.lsu.edu/cases/reporting/whalen.html

Chapter 7
Medicating Your Patients

Dispensing, Monitoring, and Managing Patients' Medications

"Mistakes are a fact of life. It is the response to error that counts"

Nikki Giovanni American poet, essayist, children's author, and editor

Maria is a 58-year old school administrator who lost her husband three years ago, and whose children each live over 500 miles away. Maria suffers from hypertension and asthma. Although she makes a good salary and has health insurance, she is worried about her ability to cope with and pay for her chronic illnesses over time. Maria has confidence in her primary care doctor. However, she feels that she is not fully informed about the long-term effects of the medications she is taking and admits that she does not always get all of her questions answered in the short time that her health plan allots for an office visit. Although she knows how to use the Internet, she is uneasy about the healthcare information she reads on the various Web sites she has visited.

Medication Error

Years ago patients would see the doctor and would be closely followed for one or two prescribed medications. Adverse interactions were rare. Today many people over the age of 50 are taking at least four or five medications and many could be taking up to 15 different drugs daily. Over 3.5 billion prescriptions are filled annually in the United States, from among 20,000 prescription drugs to choose from. Given the size of these numbers, it is not surprising that medication error is one of the most pressing concerns that doctors, medical institutions, and patients face in healthcare. The Institute of Medicine reports that medication errors injure or kill over 1.5 million people annually. These critical mistakes are preventable and involve both prescription drugs, and over the counter products, including vitamins, minerals, or herbal supplements. Errors occur in all steps of the medication process. The causes include the following:

N.B. Finn and W.F. Bria, *Digital Communication in Medical Practice,*
DOI: 10.1007/978-1-84882-355-6_8, © Springer-Verlag London Limited 2009

1. Prescribing errors – This happens at the point of care when healthcare professionals send handwritten prescriptions to the pharmacy that are illegible, resulting in misinterpretation of the actual medication or the dosage when the order is transcribed. Prescribing errors also happen when there is incomplete information among a team of healthcare professionals caring for a particular patient.
2. Drug-handling errors when full strength medications must be diluted for different applications.
3. Drug dispensing errors where the wrong medication is given to the patient.
4. Packaging and labeling errors, when drugs with similar names, abbreviations, or packaging are confused. Look alike and sound alike drug names cause one product to be mistaken for another. The use of abbreviations for drug names can result in the wrong medication or an incorrect dose given to a patient.
5. Adherence when patients do not follow instructions or choose to discontinue their medication, or are so confused by the instructions on the packaging of their prescription that they really do not know how to take the drug.
6. Human error that just happens particularly among healthcare workers who work long hours under highly stressful conditions.

Medical error is a double-edged sword. On one side is the healthcare professional whose bad handwriting causes a prescribing error, or the healthcare institution that makes a mistake; on the other side is the patient who is given a medication with directions on how to administer it, but either does not understand the directions, or does not bother to follow them. Clearly the onus is on the healthcare industry to initiate programs that resolve the causes of medical error, including: use of bar codes, e-prescribing and computer physician order entry systems, better naming conventions and packaging, and new ways to communicate with patients to help them understand how to manage and maintain their medication regimen.[1]

Electronic Prescribing (E-Prescribing)

Case Scenario #1

Karen is a 63-year-old woman with hypertension, and high blood pressure. She developed a sinus infection and went to see the doctor who checked her paper chart and handed her a prescription for an antibiotic. When she went to the pharmacy to fill the prescription, she learned that her health plan will not cover what the doctor prescribed. While Karen waited, the pharmacist called the doctor and they agreed on an alternative medication. Karen went home, took her first dose of the medication, and became very nauseous. She called her doctor in the morning and he prescribed a different antibiotic, which made her very dizzy. As a result Karen fell, broke her hip, and was hospitalized.

If Karen's doctor had access to electronic prescribing and Karen's electronic health record, he might have known if a particular drug was unacceptable to her health plan. He would also have been able to determine whether the medications that he prescribed might cause an interaction that explained the nausea. He would have instructions for follow up blood tests to determine whether the drugs being prescribed might cause any toxicity.[2]

Case Scenario #2

Ellen is a 50-year-old woman who takes six different medications for mild depression, reflux disease, and chronic asthma. At her annual visit Ellen and her doctor review her medications. The doctor makes adjustments and with a new e-prescribing system sends Ellen's prescriptions directly to a pharmacy located a couple of blocks from her home. A half hour later, Ellen picks up her medications packaged with comprehensive instructions. She asks the pharmacist a couple of questions and leaves feeling completely informed about what she has to take, when, and how often.

Prescribing medication is the physician's most frequently used tool for addressing patient problems, because it is effective in combating and ameliorating disease and other conditions. The proper or improper use of drugs has profound effect on patient outcomes. Most physicians write a prescription on a pad of paper and hand it to the patient who is directed to go to a pharmacy and fill the prescription. There is little time left during the office visit to discuss the impact and side effects of the medication. As a result the patients must learn about their medications from the written informational sheet supplied by the pharmacy. This process is inefficient and error-prone.

With the introduction of computers into the physician practice, e-prescribing is a viable substitute for the paper prescription. E-Prescribing is defined as entering a prescription into an automated data entry system (handheld, PC, or other) and generating a prescription electronically. It is based on computing technology that has the capability to enter, modify, review, and communicate drug prescriptions between the doctor or nurse practitioner and the pharmacist. In more sophisticated e-prescribing systems, the computer uses its built-in clinical decision support to check on what medications are currently being taken by the patient, whether or not the medication is covered by a patient's health plan; what possible drug–drug interactions might occur among the medications; whether or not the dosage is appropriate; whether or not the patient has a history of allergies to anything in the drug being prescribed and any other factors that are relevant in the administration of the medication. When the patient arrives at the pharmacy to pick up a prescription, detailed instructions on how to take the medication are included. E-Prescribing speeds the process of dispensing medication and provides the cross communication among doctor, pharmacist, and the patient for safer medical practice. It also helps control costs.

There are approximately 550,000 practicing physicians in the United States who are licensed to prescribe medications, yet by 2008, less than 1 in 5 were transmitting prescriptions electronically. As a response to this slow adoption of a technology that is guaranteed to save lives, the National E-Prescribing Patient Safety Initiative (NEPSI) was formed with the goal of providing free e-prescribing software to every physician in the United States, especially to individual practitioners and small groups. Challenges to the implementation of e-prescribing include the cost of the hardware and software customization, training, maintenance, and upgrades; change management in workflow around prescribing medication to patients; connectivity to multiple pharmacies and pharmacy benefit managers and maintenance of dual systems since controlled substance prescriptions cannot be sent electronically. These challenges add another layer of complexity to a physician's already overburdened practice. But they are essential. In an attempt to further the deployment of e-prescribing, some payer organizations including some of the Blues and Medicare are offering financial incentives to physicians who adopt e-prescribing technology.

Performance of an e-prescribing system over time depends on three factors:

1. The quality and validity of the knowledge base underlying the e-prescribing system at any given point in time
2. The quality and reliability of the software system applying the knowledge base to a patient's clinical condition for prescribing purposes
3. The quality, methods, and schedule for updates of both the knowledge base and the software

A March 2008 survey of 309 health IT professionals by the Healthcare Information and Management Systems Society (HIMSS) (see Figure 7.1) found that 65% of health IT professionals said that reducing the risk of medication errors is the biggest benefit to providers who use electronic prescribing. Twenty-one percent of respondents said gaining access to patients' medication histories was the biggest benefit of e-prescribing to providers, while 7% said reducing potential for fraud and tampering was the biggest benefit.

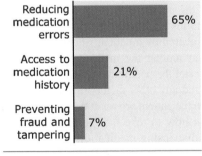

Figure 7.1 What is the biggest benefit to providers who use E-Prescribing © Health Information Management Systems Society (HIMSS)

E-prescribing has proven its value in reducing healthcare costs, bringing efficiency, and quality to medical practice and reducing medication error on a grand scale.

Patient Information and Collaborative Drug Therapy

At pharmacies throughout the nation, prescriptions have been in electronic data format for more than a decade. However, pharmacy systems only determine whether or not a prescription written by the physician is covered by the patient's health plan, and the copayment. They are not for the purpose of checking drug interactions or correcting mistakes due to illegible handwriting. E-prescribing together with EHRs and CPOE now provide the pharmacist with a complete picture of a patient's health history and enable pharmacists to work collaboratively with physicians to determine which drugs to use, what the dosages should be, and what else the patient is taking that might not interact well.

Approximately, 25% of medication errors result because patient drug information is not available during drug prescribing, dispensing, and administration. There is a severe shortage of primary care physicians (the numbers have fallen more than 50% from 1997 to 2005) resulting in an increased patient load and less time to spend with each patient discussing the particulars of medication management. Patients also shop around for doctors and specialists with the results that there is not adequate coordination of care. The patient might be on several medications with no one gatekeeper overseeing the various treatments.[3]

One solution is to have pharmacists who know exactly what medications are being taken, and how they interact provide counseling to patients, in collaboration with the patient's physician. Pharmacists can provide patients with tips on medication safety. They have the skills to evaluate patients' medication regimens relative to their disease status. They can make suggestions to the physician about additional or different medications that patients might benefit from; eliminate duplication in therapy when patients are taking more than one drug with the same ingredients; screen for drug–drug interactions, and assess patient adherence to medication. For each prescription dispensed, the pharmacist can double check, at the point of care, that the right medication is being dispensed to the right individual. The pharmacist can also review the directions on how to take the medication with the patient or the patient's designated person and can provide valuable education about prescription and nonprescription drugs that might not be safe. With the pharmacist and the physician working as a team, there is better communication among all the stakeholders in this process.[4]

Jim is a 55-year old corporate executive who spends nearly 50% of his work time traveling around the world. Jim suffers from chronic diabetes and hypertension and is on insulin therapy as well as other pills to keep his conditions under control. Although Jim has good healthcare coverage and a primary care physician that he has confidence in, Jim's busy schedule and that of his physician often does not allow time for the proper analysis and treatment reviews that his health warrants.

As a result, Jim turns to his pharmacist for advice and assistance. Daily he uploads to his computer his blood sugar measurements and the amount of insulin he delivers to himself. He then downloads that information, from wherever he is, to a pharmacist in his hometown. The pharmacist checks these measurements and confers with Jim via phone or email. They connect easily as the pharmacist is in one place and more available than Jim's PCP. Together Jim and the pharmacist agree on adjustments or changes that are needed. If there is a problem they cannot resolve, the pharmacist will check with Jim's physician.

Legislation in 41 states expands the role of pharmacists to manage drug therapy in collaboration with physicians, including: adjusting the strength and frequency of a drug regiment, administrating and ordering of some lab and diagnostic tests, modifying and reviewing medications and devices as well as advising on the hazards and uses of drugs and devices. With e-prescribing, pharmacists and providers are able to communicate quickly and efficiently, facilitating requests for new or additional medication. A Federal law, passed in the 1970s requires nursing homes to have a pharmacist review patient charts once a month to determine what medications might be causing problems. Many employers who self-insure are using pharmacist-consultants to review medications for employees with chronic conditions, because they know that this review saves them money. It seems that the logical next step should be to make collaborative drug therapy universal.[5]

Hospital Policies

At the very top of the list of ways to combat medical error are hospital policies that are not best practices. Too many errors are made when in-hospital pharmacies stock drugs improperly, nurses do not double-check to make sure they are dispensing the proper medication or doctors' bad handwriting results in the wrong drug being administered. Other errors occur when the hospital pharmacy substitutes a generic formula that could be slightly different enough to cause a problem, or when medication orders to transition a patient from intravenous to oral medication are not accurately followed. Highly publicized cases in which three babies died after receiving an overdose of the same drug, offer a vivid illustration of the problems hospitals face. In these cases, nurses mistakenly administered a concentration of heparin 1,000 times higher than intended, giving the patients a dose with a concentration of 10,000 units per milliliter instead of the correct dosage of 10 units per milliliter. The confusion was in the packaging. The packaging of the 10,000-unit dose of heparin looks very similar to that of the 10-unit dose. In both cases, each hospital received the drug from Illinois-based Baxter Healthcare Corp. In the wake of the deaths, Baxter has repackaged heparin to make the different doses more distinct, including adding a large "red alert" symbol on the more concentrated dose. With the proven technologies now available to fight these problems, many hospitals have moved prescription order writing from the physician's illegible hand to the computer. They have also instituted barcodes with a check system, where a barcode on the medication container is matched with a bar code on the patient's wrist band. These bar code systems assist healthcare providers in insuring that the right drug is administered to the patient in the right amount and at the right time.

McLeod Regional Medical Center, a 460-bed not-for-profit regional Medical Center in Florence S.C. instituted a bar code system in 2006. With this system, nurses scan the code on the badge on every patient's wristband and on every drug container to ensure the right drug is administered in the right dose to the right patient. The hospital also instituted a drug reconciliation plan that begins with a computerized patient admission assessment history form that is filled out by a nurse when the patient arrives at the hospital. The physician reviews this medication list and is able to continue or change the medications that the patient had been taking. This electronic form is then passed along to the pharmacist for verification, cutting transcription errors to nearly zero. The process is repeated anytime the patient changes location or level of care within the hospital. The final step of the reconciliation is providing each patient with complete and accurate medication information on discharge. As a result of these changes, McLeod Regional Medical Center has experienced a 90% reduction in adverse events.[6]

Brigham and Women's Hospital in Boston also eliminated prescription orders written by hand and transitioned their physicians to writing their orders on the computer, which automatically checks the request against the patient's medical history. If there is any evidence that the patient could be allergic to the drug, the computer raises a red flag. The system looks at the start and stop dates of a medication being given to a patient and sends a warning if it is time for the medication to be discontinued. Brigham and Women's Hospital has transitioned prescriptions orders from paper to a bar code system as well. The investment cost the hospital $10 million dollars, and they have seen an 85% reduction in medication errors.[7]

Confusion in the Naming of Drugs

In the hurried tense hospital environment where individuals are typically overworked, drugs that are not carefully labeled or packaged in a distinctive way can be mistaken for one another and can cause a fatal error. Name confusion among drugs is a common cause of drug-related errors. The U.S. Food and Drug Administration (FDA), is mandated by legislation to evaluate and approve the sale of all prescription medications used in the United States. Medication errors which must be reported to FDA, illustrate the complexity of the system and how easy it is for an error to occur:

- A physician ordered a 260-mg preparation of Taxol for a patient. The pharmacist prepared 260 mg of Taxotere instead. Both are chemotherapy drugs used for different types of cancer and with different recommended doses. The patient died several days late, although the death could not be directly linked to the error because the patient was already severely ill.

Table 7.1 Commonly Confused Drugs

Drug 1, indication	Drug 2, indication	Drug 3, indication
Celebrex, arthritis	**Celexa,** depression	
Clozapine, both used to treat schizophrenia but with vastly different dosages	**Olanzapine,** both used to treat schizophrenia but with vastly different dosages	
Flomax, enlarged prostrate	**Volmax,** bronchospasm	
Keppra, adults epilepsy	**Kaletra,** HIV infection	
Lamictal (lamotrigine) epilepsy	**Lamisil** (terbinafine) nail infections	
Ludiomil (maprotiline) depression	**Lomotil** (diphenoxylate) diarrhea	
Methadone, narcotic addiction	**Methylphenidate,** attention deficit disorders	
Serzone, antidepressant	**Seroquel,** schizophrenia	
Taxotere (docetaxel), chemotherapy	**Taxol** (paclitaxel), chemotherapy	
Zantac, heartburn	**Zyrtec,** allergies	**Zyprexa,** mental conditions

- Another patient died because 20 units of insulin was abbreviated as "20 U," but the "U" was mistaken for a "zero." As a result, a dose of 200 units of insulin was accidentally injected.[8]

Unfortunately, the pharmaceutical industry and the FDA have allowed a massive problem to develop when names were chosen and approved for prescription drugs (see Table 7.1). For example, the antiepileptic drug Lamictal and the antifungal drug Lamisil are so close that pharmacists have been known to misread a doctor's instructions and issue the wrong drug. Epileptic patients receiving the antifungal drug could experience continuous seizures and patients erroneously receiving the drug for epilepsy might experience rash, blood pressure changes, and other serious side effects. Errors also occur in prescribing the arthritis drug Celebrex, the anticonvulsant Cerebhyx, and the antidepressant Celexa to name just a couple of examples.[9]

Abbreviations, acronyms, dose designations, and other symbols used in prescribing medication also elevate the potential for serious problems. Pharmaceutical companies have so much equity in a drug's name, once it is on the market; there is little chance that there will ever be a complete overhaul of drug names among medications currently available. This underscores the need for better systems to check a patient's symptoms or disease against the drug being administered.

Adherence

Caroline is a 60-year old woman who loves to cook and spend time with her granddaughter. She suffers from high blood pressure and diabetes. Caroline sees her doctor every three months and fills the prescriptions he gives her at a local pharmacy. However, she readily admits that she does not remember to take her blood pressure medication unless she develops a headache. She also seeks the advice of a homeopathic consultant for herbal remedies that she believes will keep her healthy. She does not always tell her doctor about those over-the-counter products she takes.

One of the most pressing problems leading to medication error is the problem of patients who simply do not follow their physician's orders regarding their prescribed medications. This nonadherence is a problem of enormous proportions. Over 50% of individuals taking medication do not or are unable to take their medication correctly. Many people stop a prescription before completing it under the misconception that if they feel better, they no longer need it. Self-diagnosis, along with a failure to communicate with the physician lead to countless problems, and inevitably the patient returns to the physician's office with the same symptoms they had before they started the medication.[10]

The New England Journal of Medicine reported in 2005 between 33 and 69% of medication-related hospital admissions in the US were due to poor medication adherence with a resultant cost to the American public of over $100 billion a year. The article indicated that among patients with chronic conditions, adherence to a medication regimen drops radically after six months. Among patients taking antidepressants, over half of them stop taking the drugs three months after the initiation of therapy. The reasons that people fail to take prescribed medication correctly include: forgetfulness, confusion about how to take a medication, unwillingness or inability to assume the cost of the prescription, concerns about potential adverse reactions, previous experience with adverse reaction to medications, lack of information or understanding about how to use a specific remedy.[11]

Richard Carmona, the US Surgeon General from 2002 to 2006 says the more medications an individual is prescribed the larger the problem becomes. Dr. Carmona blames the lack of adherence on the "complexity of health information." "Americans are overwhelmed," he says. "We have hit a point of information overload. This is of great concern when it comes to making sure a patient knows how to use prescription drugs safely and effectively. This problem is compounded by prescription medication information that reads more like legal disclaimers than useful or actionable health information."[12]

A patient may go to the doctor and be diagnosed with a simple virus and a cough and walk away with three different medications and the instructions about how to take each, when to take each, how to separate taking the different medications, which ones need to be taken with food, etc. These instructions can often be so confusing that the wrong dosage and medication is taken at the wrong time. It is clear that when physicians and patients work together to map out a treatment patients follow the directions and have more success in controlling their illness, especially chronic disease.

Table 7.2 Guidelines to Help Patients Manage Medication

1. Make sure the patient knows what the medication is and how to spell the name which should be clearly printed on the label of each container.
2. Make sure the patient understands the dose prescribed and how often they should take the medication.
3. Insist that your patients keep a list of all medications with them at all times, or have access to a list that might be kept online.
4 Be sure that the patient understands why they are taking a medication – both prescription drugs and over the counter drugs.
5. Review medications annually with patients. This will help determine whether or not they still need everything on the list. Insist that if you agree to discontinue a medication that the patient will throw away any remaining pills when they return to their home.
6. Develop a plan of action if the patient experiences a severe side effect. Work with the patient to provide them with a process to get immediate assistance if they feel they are in a crisis situation from a medication.
7. Help patients learn where to get reliable information on over the counter and herbal medicines.
8. Encourage patients to use one pharmacy that will maintain an electronic record of all that patient's medications. This database can check for any drug interactions and help the patient better monitor and manage prescriptions.
9. Encourage patients to use a system for taking medications. The cheapest and most efficient are the pillboxes labeled for each day of the week so that a missed dose can be immediately spotted.
10. Be sure patients understand what to do if they miss a dose.
11. Encourage patients never to stop taking a medicine on their own and to be proactive.
12. Try to get patients to let you know if the cost of a medication is going to be prohibitive and work with them to seek alternatives.

Online Pharmacies

For a sizeable group of people, especially those in their 20s and 30s, making a personal choice on what drugs to take, without the benefit of a doctor's advice, and sharing medication among friends is common practice. Although these individuals claim to research drug interactions, they rely on their friend's experiences or an advertisement when it comes to popping a pill for fatigue, anxiety, or depression. They also order medications from the Internet without prescriptions. Clearly they get the message that street drugs, such as crack cocaine and heroin, are bad. But when it comes to FDA-approved pills, they think they can control their use and misuse. Patients also turn to the Internet to avoid the high cost of medications obtained through normal channels. On the Internet they can do price comparisons and find discounted drugs.[13]

Diane, 87, lives alone in a small home in Burbank Iowa. Although she is mobile and able to care for herself, she suffers from diabetes and hypertension and requires five medications daily to keep her healthy. Her doctor arranged to have her order and manage her prescriptions through a state licensed online service that has a digital copy of her medication profile, insurance information and conditions and allergies. An online pharmacist communicates with Diane by phone and email, and she is able to ask questions and access resources that he recommends. All of her pharmaceutical products are mailed to her so she does not have to leave her home.

Online pharmacies provide an invaluable service to patients who are elderly, disabled, or live in remote areas. The downside of this trend is that some health Web sites are reputable and reliable, while others are outright scams. In late 2005, US Federal drug investigators shut down 4,600 illegal Internet pharmacy sites and arrested 18 people who ran them from locations across the country. Many of these sites purport to offer prescriptions by legitimate doctors following "safe and secure" online diagnoses that typically take the form of a short questionnaire. The scam sites lead the unwary subscriber to believe that their health form is reviewed by a physician before being sent on to a pharmacist who fills the prescription. In reality many of the Web sites fill the orders or send them to an illegal wholesaler without any healthcare professional involved. Customers, rather than saving money by using these online Web services, were paying $400 for drugs that would have cost $40 with a legal prescription.[14]

There are ways for American citizens to save money on their prescription medication including some online programs that are very effective. The Veterans Administration enables Veterans to refill prescriptions online as a part of the VA's MytHealtheVet service. Five states: Illinois, Kansas, Wisconsin, Vermont, and Missouri have implemented an online drug program I-SaveRx that allows citizens to purchase cheaper, safe prescription drugs from state-approved pharmacies in the US, Europe, and Canada. With the exception of these few programs, there are many hazards to online medication purchases that the unwary consumer might not understand. Physicians should refer their patients to the FDA Website where there are guidelines regarding the use of online prescription fulfillment services at http://www.fda.gov/buyonline.

Table 7.3 lists FDA guidelines regarding online prescription fulfillment.

Table 7.3 FDA Guidelines Regarding Online Prescription Fulfillment

1.	Website requires a prescription.
2.	Website has licensed pharmacists on staff to answer your questions
3.	Website is licensed by the state board of pharmacy (check: http://www.nabp.info for a list.)
4.	Website sells only drugs approved by the FDA and will openly tell you what organization you are dealing with.
5.	Website does not ask for identifiable information especially a social security number.

Direct-to-Consumer Advertising

Steve had just finished an exhausting week at work and was very tired and kind of depressed. When his friend Dave offered him a Ritalin that he had left over from medication that he never finished, Steve, who had heard all about Ritalin from an advertisement he saw on television, popped the medication in his mouth and went along for a night on the town with Alan and Katie. Alan was feeling anxious so Katie offered him an Ativan, which he readily accepted, having read about it in a magazine on men's health.

Direct-to-consumer (DTC) advertising has become a leading form of marketing practiced by pharmaceutical companies to promote new prescription medications. Overwhelmingly positive advertising claims presented on television and in magazine advertisements often result in inappropriate demands for new drugs by patients. The FDA is charged with regulating the promotion of prescription drugs including the content of DTC advertising as legislated in the Federal Food Drug and Cosmetic Act (FFDCA). The act sets general standards that require that the advertisements present accurate information and fairly represent both the benefits and the risks of advertised drugs. However, this is difficult to regulate. The pharmaceutical industry spends upwards of $5 billion annually on the marketing of drugs. Survey results published in the February 2007 issue of Consumer Reports magazine reveal that 78% of primary care physicians are asked by their patients for specific drugs they have seen advertised on television. Much of the ease with which Americans imbibe prescription medication is due to DTC advertising. Patients who are bombarded with positive messages about the benefits of pills for depression, anxiety, cholesterol, and high blood pressure begin to believe those messages and feel that it is safe and effective to use these drugs.

Resources for Safe Healthcare and Medication Advice

1. FDA – MedWatch – The FDA's safety information and adverse event reporting program. 1-800-332-1088 http://www.fda.gov/medwatch/how.htm2.
2. Institute for Safe Medication Practices – This organization accepts reports from consumers and health professionals related to medication. They publish Safe Medicine, a consumer newsletter on medication errors.
   1800 Bayberry Rd., Suite 810 Huntingdon Valley, PA 19006-3520, 215-947-7797, http://www.ismp.org/Pages/Consumer.html
3. U.S. Pharmacopeia (www.usp.org) is an official public standards-setting authority for all prescription and over-the-counter medicines and other health care products manufactured or sold in the United States.
4. MedMARX an anonymous medication error reporting program used by hospitals. 12601 Twinbrook Parkway Rockville, MD 20852,1-800-822-8772, http://www.medmarx.com
5. National Association of Boards of Pharmacy http://www.nabp.net

Key Points

1. There are so many prescriptions written annually that medication error has become a problem of major proportions. The fault lies with both the healthcare professional and the patient. The solution is complex involving several issues including: prescribing errors, hospital procedures, naming and labeling of drugs, patient adherence, and human error.

2. Electronic Prescribing is one of the proven ways that medications errors have been reduced. With electronic prescribing the issue of illegible handwritten prescriptions is eliminated. E-Prescribing also helps to eliminate drug-drug interaction and overdosing and fosters cross communication among the team working on finding the right medication for the patient.

3. With an increase in the number of patients with chronic conditions who need monitoring and a decrease in the number of medical school graduates going into primary care, one solution is to involve the pharmacist in a collaborative relationship with the physician to help answer patients' questions about their medications and help monitor and manage medications. Pharmacists are also well positioned to check on patient adherence.

4. Too many medication errors occur in the hospital. A change in the way medication is labeled, stocked, and dispensed can resolve some of these issues through the implementation of computer physician order entry and bar code systems.

5. Naming of drugs has got to be more efficiently handled and monitored because name confusion is a common cause of drug-related errors. It is a given that there are too many drugs on the market whose names are so similar that they can easily be confused. The pharmaceutical industry is not going to change their naming systems so the healthcare industry has to put more rigid checks in place to offset this problem. This might include larger warnings and notations on labels to clearly indicate what a drug is to be used for. This, in combination with the bar code systems, can help the nurses who administer these medications.

6. There needs to be better communication between physicians and patients to foster adherence to prescribed medications. Patients need to understand the reasons for the medication in the first instance and understand the consequences if the medication treatment plan agreed upon is not followed.

7. Online pharmacies can serve a valuable purpose, particularly for individuals who are homebound or live in remote areas and are unable to access their medication unless it is sent through the mail. However, as with everything on the Web, there are good and bad Web sites and patients need to be coached in how to distinguish among them.

8. DTC advertising of drugs by pharmaceutical companies, retail pharmacies, and distributors contributes to the confusion about medication. Physicians need to clarify for their patients what is beneficial and what is harmful to them, and urge their patients to put more trust in their advice than in the advertisements they read and see.

References and Notes

1. Preventing Medication Errors, National Academies Press July, 2006
2. Adapted from a case cited in the Report of the Join Clinical Decision Support Workgroup, March 2005 "Clinical Decision Support in Electronic Prescribing: Recommendations and Action Plan," sponsored by the Office of the National Coordinator for Health Information Technology (ONCHIT) at the Department of Health and Human Services (HHS)
3. *Study of Factors Influencing Medical Students in Their Choice of Family Practice as a Specialty - Arizona Study.* Conducted by Janet H. Senf, Ph.D., Doug Campos-Outcalt, M.D., M.P.A., and Randa Kutob, M.D. Department of Family and Community Medicine, University of Arizona www.aafp.org)
4. "Protecting U.S. Citizens from Inappropriate Medication Use, Institute for Safe Medication Practices, White Paper 2007
5. www.aacp.org *"The Druggist is in"* by Elizabeth Agnvail, the Washington Post, December 14, 2004.
6. www.modernhealthcare.com, "How we Cut Drug Errors" by Natasha Nicol and Leanne Huminski, August 28, 2006.
7. Rosemary Gibson and Janardan Prasad Singh, *Wall of Silence* Lifeline Press, Washington D.C. 2003 (Also reported in www.federaltelemedicine.com/n022205.htmand story in bostgonbizjournals.com "Lines are drawn to Stop Drug-Dispensary Errors" by Mark aHoller April 5–11 2005)
8. www.fda.gov
9. www.fda.gov/fdacx/features/2000/500+err.html
10. *HealthMedia Moving Beyond Traditional Approaches to C&P,* Kevin Wildenhaus, Ph. D.
11. Osterberg L, Blaschike T. Drug therapy adherence to medication. *New England Journal of Medicine* 2005
12. Carmona RH. Health literacy: a national priority. *Journal of General Internal Medicine* 2006;21:803.
13. Amy Harmon, *"Young and Assured and Playing Pharmacist to Friends,"* New York Times, Nov. 16, 2005
14. New York Times October 24 2005 *Pharmacies Endorse Crackdown on Fraud* by Bob Tedeschi) www.nytimes.com/2005

Chapter 8
All About Money

Mary was an accountant, working for one of the large national accounting firms. She loved her job and never took a sick day in the 13 years she had been with the company. She had not even bothered to find a doctor who accepted her insurance plan. At age 35 Mary was diagnosed with Lupus, a disease in which the immune system attacks healthy tissue. Her disease progressed rapidly and soon she was unable to work. Several visits to her doctors, a seizure which sent her to the emergency room, high doses of expensive medications, a requirement for CAT scans every six weeks to monitor her disease resulted in mounting bills that her insurance company began to question and eventually stopped paying. Although lupus can be fatal, many people who have it live a normal life span, according to the Lupus Foundation of America. The disease is usually managed with appropriate medication. However, when insurance companies refuse to pay and individuals deplete their own resources, the medications and the treatments stop.

Mary was a fiercely proud woman. When the payments stopped, she stopped seeing her doctors and stopped getting tests that would monitor her disease and prevent even more insidious events. She turned to the government for assistance but the State Medicaid bureaucracy was merely another maze to wander through which was overwhelming to Mary. She became depressed and refused to seek further assistance. Two years after her diagnosis, Mary died of complications.

How We Measure Healthcare Costs

For decades the American medical establishment separated money from medical care on the premise that treating patients should not be tainted by financial considerations. During that era the business proposition between doctors and patients was simply that the patient paid the physician in exchange for the doctor's advice and skill–fee for service. As the cost of care climbed, economic realities forced changes in the system. It seemed that fee-for-service payment would induce doctors to order more tests and to hospitalize patients more frequently than other payment methods. Managed care was introduced, creating an environment where money suddenly

N.B. Finn and W.F. Bria, *Digital Communication in Medical Practice*,
DOI: 10.1007/978-1-84882-355-6_9, © Springer-Verlag London Limited 2009

played a major role in clinical decisions. It was thought that managed care would provide better services for insured patients, while controlling costs. However, contractual agreements inherent in the managed care configuration results in financial pressure on doctors to do less in every aspect of patient care including: how long a doctor spends with a patient during an annual office visit; what diagnostic tests are ordered; which of several beneficial therapies are deployed; which drugs are prescribed. HMOs typically do not pay for a more comprehensive visit, sometimes penalizing the healthcare professional for doing what needs to be done and for being thorough. With the HMO system patients must get prior approval for tests, labs, and referrals to specialists, so clinical decisions are not always made by the doctor, but are subject to the rules set by the HMO. In spite of all this economizing, when the results are tallied and the evaluations are completed it becomes obvious that managed care has not managed to control costs, nor has it resulted in higher quality care. In fact, managed care discourages doctors from practicing the high quality professional standards that they brought to their medical practice.

By the beginning of the twenty-first century, US health spending continued to outpace inflation rising at 7% annually. In 2008, health spending was over $1.9 trillion or $5 billion a day – over 15% of the Gross Domestic Product (as seen in Figure 8.1). These numbers include government expenditures through Medicaid and Medicare, private health insurance, and out of pocket expenditures. Part of the spending problem in American medicine lies in the belief among American citizens

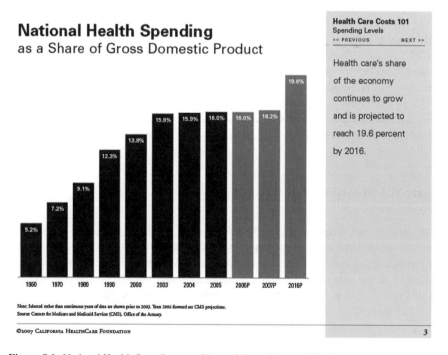

Figure 8.1   National Health Spending as a Share of Gross Domestic Product

that healthcare is a right and not a privilege. Americans feel they should receive not only basic care but the best that medical science can provide, no matter how they may abuse their health. Although most people contribute something to the cost of care, they expect the rest to come from the insurer, the government or some other source.[1]

In his book, *Crisis of Abundance: Rethinking How We Pay for Healthcare*, author Arnold Kling, economist calls the American approach of encouraging everyone to undergo routine screening procedures; performing MRI and CT scans to rule out conditions and the typical: "heroic" efforts during the last 90 days of life "*premium medicine*." Kling explains that Americans routinely expect to be allowed to see medical specialists and avail themselves of advanced technology. He contends that although there is no hard data on whether or not this approach affects the outcome, it clearly affects the cost of healthcare. Kling compares the use of expensive medical procedures in the US with its European cousins, stating that heart bypass surgery is about three times as prevalent in the US as it is in France and twice as prevalent as in the UK. Angioplasty is more than twice as prevalent in the US as in France and about seven times as prevalent as in the UK.[2]

Twenty years ago, the protocol for a patient who came in for an annual visit might be one or two tests. With the diagnostic tools available today, the same patient can require up to 20 tests, with 30 pieces of information coming back to the doctor for analysis and decision. The result is usually a very accurate diagnosis. However, the cost of this one encounter, the subsequent tests and the sheer amount of information the doctor must interpret and integrate into a treatment plan raises the cost incrementally. Couple that with the fact that years ago a patient might be taking two medications. Advances in modern medicine are such that today the average patient can be taking as many as ten medications prescribed by a team of three or four specialists.

In a study conducted by a group of medical students at Dartmouth Medical School, data showed that in the last six months of life, patients in Oregon spend an average of eight days in the hospital, while patients in New York spend 35 days. In Oregon, the patient is seen by an average of 14 doctors; in New York 35 doctors see the patient. In the last two years of life, the average Oregon patient costs the system $25,500 and the New York patient $38,300. The study found no evidence that the New York patient enjoyed a better quality experience, reinforcing that more care is not necessarily better care, nor does it result in better long-term outcomes.[3]

The Underinsured and the Uninsured

Most Americans get health insurance through their employer, a family member who signs on with an employer-based insurance plan, or an association or other group with which they have an affiliation. The sources for health insurance coverage in the United States include employers who cover over 160 million nonelderly people, Medicaid which covers 30 million children, parents, the disabled (and in some states other adults); and another 14 million people who obtain their healthcare coverage through the direct purchase market. There are others who are covered by Medicare and military health insurance programs. Together these insurance plans extend coverage to over 210 million Americans, leaving 47 million nonelderly Americans uninsured, 8 million who are children.

A study conducted by The Commonwealth Fund (shown in Figure 8.2) found that the number of American adults who had inadequate health insurance to cover their medical expenses rose 60% from 2003 to 2007, from 16 million to more than 25 million people. Couple that with the millions of uninsured people, (these numbers range from 10 million to 50 million depending upon who is doing the counting, and whether we are in a period of full employment or a recession when people lose jobs and subsequently lose health insurance), and it is a big problem. Add in the increasing numbers of baby boomers, an elderly population that is reliant on costly prescription medication, frequent check ups, hospitalization, chronic care monitoring and extraordinary medical expenses, and the problem becomes enormous.

The system of job-based insurance that was effective during the latter half of the twentieth century does not work in the twenty-first century ehealth era. Health

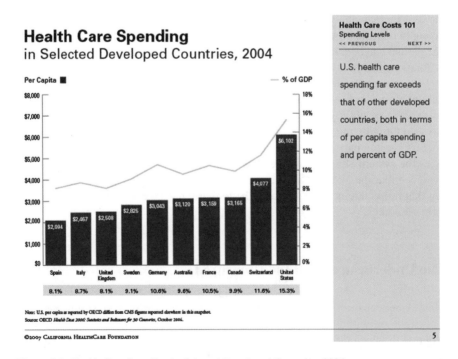

Figure 8.2 Health Care Spending in Selected Developed Countries, 2004

benefits are the most important factor in employment services, second only to wages. Employers, well aware of this, are straining to stay solvent and offer the benefits their employees need. Many have also expanded employee health benefits for wellness, convenient care, adherence, on the theory that better healthcare will lower health expenses in the long run and lead to higher work productivity. It is not easy. Starbucks Corporation spends more on health insurance for its 80,000 employees than on the raw materials needed to brew its coffee. The national grocery chain Safeway reported that the $1 billion that it spent on employee healthcare in 2006 exceeded its net income. Yet in spite of these high costs, patients in a healthcare crisis or those with chronic conditions quickly discover that their job-based healthcare coverage does not meet all of their needs and leaves them underinsured.[4]

Then there are the uninsured - *When Dan was laid off from his engineering job he lost not only his work, his income, and his feeling of self worth but his health insurance as well. Payments were out of the question as Dan did not have the resources to keep up with the premiums. Diagnosed with depression six months after the lay off and unable to find other work, Dan also lost his condo, his car, and his credit cards and ended up on the street. Having asthma all of his life, Dan began to develop breathing problems and contracted pneumonia. He landed in the emergency room of a large urban public hospital, and was admitted.*

Dan is among millions of recently uninsured American individuals who often avoid healthcare needs for so long that they precipitate into a major, sometimes life-threatening crisis. This is a syndrome that not only risks the lives of these individuals but sends healthcare costs for everyone spiraling upward, making it more difficult for the average citizen to receive the care that is needed. Dan's story is not atypical. People without health insurance have health care needs that are generally met when they end up at a publicly supported clinic or a hospital emergency room. They are treated. However, their unpaid medical bills are ultimately shifted to the taxpayer, who is already paying high premiums for their own insurance, out of pocket co-payments, and dealing with the increasing high costs of healthcare that they cannot afford.

Although healthcare costs have also risen exponentially throughout the world, other countries address the cost control issue in very different ways. Those countries with universal health insurance systems such as Canada, Great Britain, and Australia rely on organized cooperation, planning and waiting lists to contain costs. In many countries, where healthcare is controlled by the government, each doctor is paid a flat salary. This eliminates financial incentives to over-treat (although there is a risk that they will under-treat). Those systems also deploy technology to moderate expenses. They believe that every physician should use electronic health records, which they fund and provide. They also limit the total supply of healthcare professionals and decide at the government level where a doctor can practice to disburse medical services throughout the country. These systems are not without their problems, but healthcare services are spread more evenly throughout the population and everyone is covered.

Controlling Health Expenses with Information Technology

The adoption of digital communication technology has been proposed as a part of the solution to the soaring healthcare bill. Widespread adoption of electronic health records, particularly those with guidelines embedded, could help to reduce the cost of care nationwide to the tune of between $75 and $80 billion annually. These numbers are based on the premise that doctors who have electronic records are better equipped to provide efficient care: they will order fewer tests; require fewer visits from patients; and shorten their patients' time in the hospital. There is also a belief that electronic records will vastly reduce administrative costs with less paperwork for administrative assistants and nurses, and overall efficiency in providing patient care. These cost reductions come with a price - approximately $8 million annually over a 15-year period, or a total of $120 million to implement electronic health records across the nation. This sum does not take into account the additional millions of dollar required for health information exchange and telemedicine networks, the data warehouses to support true decision support for physicians and e-prescribing systems. Nor does the projected expenditure account for the healthcare professionals' time during the implementation of health information technology.

During the first decade of the twenty-first century, only a small percentage of healthcare professionals accepted and bought into the idea of digital communication technology to reduce costs and improve their profit. A Manhattan Research study reported that in 2008 only 36% of doctors communicate with patients online. A smaller percentage, approximately 25% had installed electronic health records. There are sound economic reasons why so few have systems. Among the millions of physicians who are independent practitioners or who are in small group practices, it is difficult to cost justify an electronic health record. The initiative to implement electronic health records and digital health information exchange lacks funding sources, both public and private. Until money is placed on the table nothing will change. The question is how much we, as a society, are willing to pay out today to achieve more efficient, financially viable healthcare for everyone in the future.

There are political/logistical problems that complicate the issue. Community practitioners are often on the staff of several community hospitals that do not have the same or compatible health records. Standards, although evolving, are not resolved. A national effort, early in the century, to create an information infrastructure with the ability to share health information across geographies floundered without funding by the US Congress. Many of the attempts to implement regional health information exchanges (RHIOs) have also failed, mainly due to lack of funds and a misalignment of those who financially benefit vs. those who assume the economic responsibility for implementation of the RHIO (payers vs. providers). The business case for investing in health information technology also relates to the financial effect on the healthcare organization's bottom line. For hospitals that is often negative. Studies show that a well functioning HIT system in the hospital reduces the length of stay for patients and reduces readmissions - all sources of revenue. Unquestionably, HIT with the ability to share information and avoid redundant tests and treatment does reduce the total cost of care for many patients; However, disbursing cost savings, does not solve the issue of affordable healthcare for all individuals.

Payers including private insurers such as Aetna, and Cigna, large employers, government agencies such as CMS are the entities that will realize the greatest gains from the cost efficiencies of HIT. They need to partner with health organizations including hospitals and physician groups and find ways to support HIT, including: electronic health records and computerized order entry, e prescribing, telemedicine networks health information exchange and a host of other digital communication applications. In the past, the Stark (physician self referral) rules prevented a health system from giving anything of value to a potential referral source that might induce referrals. The Medicare Modernization Act of 2003 mandated that CMS create exceptions to these rule and in August 2006, the final rule was published with two exceptions to the Stark Regulations:

1. An exception that protects certain arrangements involving electronic prescribing technology.
2. An exception that protects certain arrangements involving interoperable EHRs or information technology and training services. This exception states that any entity that furnishes CMS designated health services can offer an EHR, information technology, or training services. This includes all interoperable electronic health records, information technology, or training that is necessary and predominately pertains to the creation, maintenance, transmission, and reception of those records.

Consumer-Directed Health Plans (CDHP)

The presence of digital communications that support healthcare decision making and empower the consumer with better, more accessible information about health issues supports the concept that the burden of deciding how to spend health care dollars can be shifted from government agencies, employers, and insurers to the patient who would be responsible for deciding which health insurance benefits are important and how to purchase health services. This new wave is called Consumer-Directed Health Plans (CDHP). CDHP applies only to those who are employed and excludes the unemployed, the indigent, illegals, who are denied healthcare coverage, and those on Medicaid.

The Delaney's are a middle class American family with two young children, a modest home with a mortgage, a dog, two cars and a couple of credit cards, which always seem to have a monthly balance that is larger than the Delaney's budget for that same time period. Although both parents work and both have received "cost of living" increases over the past several years, there never seems to be enough money to make ends meet. An analysis of their budget reveals that higher payroll deductions

from Dad's paycheck for healthcare, which covers the entire family, and higher out
of pocket expenses for medical needs during those same several years has exceeded
the cost of living raises that they achieved.

The Delaney's are not unique. Their story repeats itself across the country. Two
hard-working citizens making a genuine contribution to society are financially
buried under the burden of critical healthcare expenses. Receiving adequate healthcare is unachievable for the average American family today, unless the model
changes. CDHP was devised by health policymakers who believe it is a way to
reduce healthcare costs while offering optimal healthcare coverage that meets the
patient's needs. It is based on the premise that if patients were to manage their
healthcare, they would do it more efficiently than the bureaucratic organizations
currently handling that task. CDHC is based on the patient/consumer having all the
necessary information to make informed decisions. With informed consumers driving their healthcare with cash in hand, a more competitive marketplace would
emerge. Insurers would be forced to provide more cost effective programs.
Providers would become more efficient in handling patients; Much of the overhead
and paperwork generated by the systems that adds little to society's health and well
being, and much to the cost would be controlled.

The basic configuration of CDHP includes high deductible insurance plans,
combined with a savings account option that CDHP enrollees can use to pay for
routine or extraordinary health expenses with tax-preferred funds. These programs
are supported by tools to assist enrollees in their health care decision making. There
are two basic types of savings accounts.

Health Reimbursement Accounts (HRA)

These accounts are medical care reimbursement plans established by employers
and used by employees to pay for healthcare. Employers typically commit to a
specific amount of money to be available in the Health Reimbursement Accounts
(HRA) for medical expenses. Unspent funds in an HRA are usually carried over to
the next year. However, the employee does not take the HRA balance when they
leave the job.

Health Savings Accounts (HSA)

These accounts are set up to assist patients with payment of out of pocket health
expenses. Both employees and employers can contribute to a Health Savings
Account (HSA) up to an annual amount limit determined by a statutory cap. The
employee's contributions to an HSA are made on a preincome tax basis and are
often arranged through a payroll deduction. Employees own their HSA and retain
the funds if they were to leave the job.

CDHPs only apply to those individuals who have health insurance and who can afford to set aside a sum of money for healthcare. They leave out a large portion of the population and fail to address the high cost of implementing and supporting the healthcare infrastructure with the high cost of new technology.

Pay-for-Performance (P4P)

Just as CDHPs empower consumers and get them involved in determining how to spend healthcare dollars, Pay-for-Performance (P4P) is a way to incent physicians to reduce cost and improve the quality of the care they deliver. P4P is a payment approach used in healthcare that correlates payment to how well providers adhere to practice standards and achieve certain outcomes, based on a set of performance measures. A performance measure is a set of technical specifications that define how to calculate a "rate" for some indicator of quality. The healthcare industry uses a tool, accepted by more than 90% of American health plans entitled The Healthcare Effectiveness Data and Information Set (HEDIS). HEDIS measures performance on various dimensions of care and service. For example, HEDIS defines very precisely how plans should calculate the percentage of members who should have received beta blockers against those who were actually given a prescription. Using these measures, plans can determine what their P4P rate is and how they compare with other plans. The primary areas of focus for HEDIS measures are preventive care delivery and disease management for chronic illness. Early P4P efforts focused on establishing common measure sets such as those developed by the National Committee for Quality Assurance (NCQA). NCQA developed quality standards and performance measures for a broad range of health care entities including Physician Recognition Programs: Diabetes Physician Recognition Program, Heart/ Stroke Physician Recognition Program, Physician Practice Connections and the Back Pain Recognition Program, all of which include a payment incentive.

When P4P was introduced, doctors generally were indignant. But they learned quickly that they are not the only ones graded and rewarded. Firemen, policemen, corporate management workers, and teachers are all graded and rewarded to provide quality service. The premise of P4P is a noble one. Doctors and healthcare organizations that deliver quality, efficient care, earn more money and hopefully reduce overall cost of patient care. However, the design and implementation of P4P programs are inequitable and diverse. In some P4P programs the bar is so low, that what is truly important is not what is measured. There is much work to be done to establish P4P standards before this solution fulfills its promise to reduce cost and elevate quality of healthcare delivery.

The American healthcare state of crisis stems from a misalignment of the business of healthcare impacting both the quality and the availability of healthcare for patient populations. Although as a people, Americans have been sold on the need to seek out the latest drug or technology, the result is spiraling costs and less access to the most basic care. The time definitely has come for the American healthcare system to decide whether superlative care for the few outweighs the need for access to care of the many. There is a critical need to realign in the way much of the rest of the developed world has done, behind preventative medicine and individual responsibility for health and healthy behaviors as well as choices for spending health dollars. The industry needs to look at the disparity between the dollars required to build a national health information exchange infrastructure with electronic health records, e prescribing, data warehouses and other digital technologies, and the subsequent savings as a result of having these capabilities. Physicians need to become more aggressive about controlling costs and improving quality and more open-minded about deploying health information technology. What is at stake here is the future stability of the healthcare system and its ability to provide adequate care to the maximum number of patients possible.

Key Points

1. The healthcare landscape has evolved from a focus on fee for service payment to physicians to managed care of the latter part of the twentieth century, neither of which work well to satisfy the healthcare professional and keep costs contained.
2. Healthcare costs are driven by the enormous sums that are expended to fund medical care that many American consumers have become accustomed to. With these expenditures comprising such a large portion of the Gross Domestic Product everyone involved: physicians, patients, policymakers, government officials, and large health institutions need to realize that care at higher cost is not necessarily better, safer, more effective care.
3. The employer-based insurance model has proven to be defective because in a healthcare crisis the majority of individuals with such coverage find themselves to be underinsured.
4. America also faces the issue of what to do about the uninsured and how to even out coverage even if it means less comprehensive care than the American public is accustomed to.
5. The implementation of health information technology brings efficiencies to the healthcare industry and particularly to an individual physician's practice. However, there are major hurdles to overcome with HIT, not the least of which is the cost of implementing the technology and resolving the question of who will pay.
6. Consumer Directed Health Plans (CDHP) are one way to finance health with critical involvement from the individuals/patients who must be empowered to decide how to spend their health dollars.
7. Pay for Performance is a twenty-first century initiative that provides incentives to physicians to maintain a set of standards in treating patients, particularly those with chronic illness. Over the long-term, an effective P4P program should reduce costs and increase quality and safety in patient care.

8. Solving the Healthcare cost crisis must involve a coalition of major payers, government entities, and private groups working with healthcare institutions to address the shortfall in health information technology implementation and the effort to bring back efficiency and quality to caring for the health of the nation's citizens. Payers who will gain the most should assume a large portion of this cost.

References and Notes

1. California Health Foundation Snapshot Health Care Costs 101, 2007
2. Kling Arnold. *Crisis of Abundance: Rethinking How We Pay for Health Care*. Washington D.C.: Cato Institute; 2006.
3. "Need a Knee Replaced? Check your Zip Code by Stephanie Saul, June 11 2007 NY Times www.nytimes.com/2007/0611/business/businessspecial/
4. Associated Press, September 14, 2005 www.nytimes.com/200701/25/business

Chapter 9
The Quality Quotient

Quality in primary care means thinking broadly because any
and every problem of human biology can present itself.
It means making judicious decisions with limited data about
children and adults neither overreacting not being blasé;
it means wielding one's words with precision and with a
profound appreciations of the social context of the patients.
It means, as gatekeepers, knowing where to guide patients.

(Groopman, Jerome, M.D. How Doctors Think,
Houghton Mifflin Company, Boston, NY 2007)

When he was 10-months old, Billy developed severe digestive problems. Now at
age 3, Billy has seen countless doctors, undergone innumerable tests, and has been
hospitalized twice. Nevertheless, doctors do not have a diagnosis. Each time Billy
sees a new specialist, his mother Anne has to provide a complete medical history
and a current list of his medications as there is no continuous electronic health
record for Billy that can be communicated from provider to provider.

Ironically, Billy's Dad, John, is an M.D. with a specialty in psychiatry. When
John finished his residency, the family moved from Washington State to California.
This meant yet another group of new doctors for Billy. They ordered many repeat
tests and procedures and prescribed new medications and every charge was ques-
tioned by their health insurer. The family is distraught with worry about how they
will be able to handle the cost of Billy's care, long term, and why he is not thriving
as a normal 3-year-old.

The absence of a trusted gatekeeper who is able to oversee Billy's medical issues
and direct the flow of information about Billy to various specialists; the lack of a
comprehensive medical record that can be accessed digitally by all of the doctors
taking care of Billy; the inability of the healthcare system to work with the family
to control the cost of his care; the long-term impact of not having answers to Billy's
problem, all threaten Billy's well being.

N.B. Finn and W.F. Bria, *Digital Communication in Medical Practice*,
DOI: 10.1007/978-1-84882-355-6_10, © Springer-Verlag London Limited 2009

A Broken System

The US healthcare system in the twenty-first century is broken. It is broken because the United States spends more money on healthcare than any other nation in the world – 15% of the Gross National Product - and yet, is the only industrialized nation that does not ensure that all citizens have healthcare coverage. As a result, 44 million Americans have no health insurance and 18,000 citizens die every year because they do not have the means to seek medical care. Astoundingly, in the event of a catastrophic illness, the majority of Americans are underinsured, lacking the means to pay for the medications, rehabilitation, and the long-term care required, and often forgoing treatment when the economics do not match the expectation. Compounding the problem, there are shortages of primary care physicians, medical errors at unacceptable rates, crises too often in hospital emergency rooms, unacceptable wait times for inpatient beds, and an outdated and inadequate healthcare infrastructure. The World Health Organization ranks the US healthcare system 37th among industrialized nations, between Costa Rica and Slovenia, on the basis of the infant mortality rate in the population! Although the World Health Organization may not be comparing apples to apples since the US reporting system on birth and deaths is different from other nations, this does not change the fact that the US healthcare system is so focused on managing cost that there are failures throughout the system in managing the quality of care delivered. Much to the surprise and chagrin of many in America, there are countries throughout the world where the health system works much more effectively and efficiently for their citizens.[1]

With this bleak situation in mind, the Institute of Medicine embarked on a study of quality in healthcare. In its unique report, "***Crossing the Quality Chasm***", the IOM states: "*the healthcare system is in need of fundamental change, because it is not delivering the care that the public should receive.*" The IOM researchers conclude that between the health care we have and the care we could have "***lies not just a gap but a chasm.***" This report, released in 2001, outlines the changes that must be instituted to address the failures of the healthcare system[2] (See Table 9.1)[3] and the acceptable standards of care (see Table 9.2).[4]

Table 9.1 Quality Criteria as Outlined by the Institute of Medicine[3]

1. Safe	Avoiding injuries to patients from the care that is intended to help them.
2. Effective	Providing services based on scientific knowledge to all who can benefit and refraining from providing services to those not likely to benefit.
3. Patient-centered	Providing care that is respectful of and responsive to individual patient preferences, needs, and values and ensuring that patient values guide all clinical decisions.
4. Timely	Reducing waits and sometimes harmful delays both for those who receive care and those who give care.
5. Efficient	Avoiding waste including waste of equipment, supplies, ideas, and energy.
6. Equitable	Providing care that does not vary in quality because of personal characteristics such as gender, ethnicity, geographic location, and socioeconomic status.

Table 9.2 Standards of Care as Outlined by the Institute of Medicine[4]

1. Care based on continuous healing relationships	Patients should receive care whenever they need it and in many forms, not just face-to-face visits, i.e., 24/7 care with access via the Internet, telephone, and other available means.
2. Customization based on patient needs and values	Individualized care to each patient.
3. The patient as the source of control	Patients need to be given the necessary information and the opportunity to exercise the degree of control they choose over healthcare decisions that affect them.
4. Shared knowledge and free flow of information	Patients should have unfettered access to their medical information and to clinical knowledge. Clinicians and patients need to communicate effectively and share information.
5. Evidence-based decision making	Care based on the best scientific knowledge available.
6. Safety as a system property	Safe for all patients, in all of its processes, all the time. In a safe system patients need to tell caregivers something only once.
7. Transparency	A health care system that makes information available to patients and their families and, in turn, allows them to make informed decisions, while at the same time respecting confidentiality.
8. Anticipation of needs	A healthcare system that anticipates patients needs rather than simply reacting to events.
9. Value	Care that does not waste the patient's or care giver's time and money.
10. Cooperation	An environment that fosters communication among clinicians and is patient-centric.

Why Quality is so Hard to Achieve

Quality in healthcare is one of those philosophical capstones that everyone espouses and nobody knows quite how to achieve. In looking at the IOM standards of care, it is immediately apparent that patient centric care based on open and complete disclosure of information is key. This is not easily achieved in an environment where healthcare professionals use their best diagnostic skills to address what is obvious, but do not have the tools to evaluate every possibility. Safe patient care is also difficult to achieve in the high stress work environment of the twenty-first century with a healthcare worker who is often underpaid, overworked, and tired.

Health Information Technology

The physician–patient partnership where information including medical records is shared and problems are addressed dynamically is a new phenomenon in US healthcare. Success of this partnership depends upon the deployment of those digital technologies outlined in previous chapters. The IOM recommendations are very specific on this point. The technologies include:

1. **Electronic Health Records** where information on a patient is held digitally in a computer file accessible by all of the patient's providers in a particular institution with the patient's permission.
2. **Electronic Communication** between patients and their physicians, using communication channels that are available 24/7, including email and patient portals, to reduce unnecessary face visits and enable physicians to provide quick responses to patients' nonemergency questions and concerns.
3. **Electronic Prescribing** that provides up to date formulary information at the time a physician writes a prescription and facilitates electronic transmission of a legible prescription to the pharmacy where an electronic record of all of the patient's medications is available to help prevent drug–drug and food–drug interaction issues.
4. **Ambulatory computerized physician order entry systems** that facilitate physician orders at the point of care for medications, laboratory tests, and procedures.
5. **Inpatient CPOE**, which reduces record-keeping errors in the hospital setting.
6. **Regional Data Sharing and Health Information Exchange** that coordinates patient data across a geographical area when patients are seen at multiple provider sites.
7. **Deployment of the e-ICU** where the limited number of intensivists available work as a team to remotely monitor several intensive and critical care units within a hospital or a regional hospital system. This insures that every ICU and CCU patient has the benefit of the intensivist's expertise.
8. **Online Tools** to support disease management applications for patients with chronic conditions that require patient involvement; tools that enable patients to take more responsibility for understanding and managing their health.
9. **Personal health records** where patients assume responsibility for keeping accurate and timely health records that are shared with all of their healthcare professionals. These PHRs take many forms including those supported by various payers and those offered by Google Health and Microsoft Healthvault.
10. **Portals** where patients are able to schedule appointments, update their records, retrieve their lab results, review their prescriptions, and send secure messages to their healthcare professionals or engage in a Web visit.
11. **Web Visits** where patients are able to talk with their physician to resolve nonemergency issues without having to leave their home or office.
12. **Telemedicine** the use of communication technology such as video and audio conferencing, scanning devices, monitoring equipment, high bandwidth channels, and the Internet to enable medical consults when distance separates patients from their healthcare professionals.

There is no question that a direct benefit of health IT (see Figure 9.1) is operational efficiencies including the reduction of administrative and clerical error. However, the real gains from IT deployment are improvements in systems of care

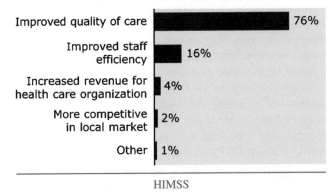

Figure 9.1 What would be the biggest benefit of clinicians using IT? © Health Information Management Systems Society (HIMSS)

including the ability to have all pertinent information on a patient in one place, available to all healthcare professionals involved in that patient's care via an electronic record that is transmittable across facilities, regions, or nations. It is this interoperability that enables healthcare professionals to make care decisions specifically tailored to the needs, preferences, and medical challenges of each individual they are charged with caring for. Combining the availability of the health record with computerized order entry, the extensive digital databases and online resources now available, the physician is able to make decisions based on best practices that not only impact the individual patient but also positively impact a larger patient population. The availability of electronic communication 24/7 provides constant, uninterrupted care, and control in ordinary and emergency situations and free flow of information between patient and healthcare professional. The resources of the Internet provide shared knowledge, and, with proper guidance from healthcare professionals, enable patients to become informed, equal partners in their care.[5]

Evidence-Based Healthcare Delivery

The presence of technology raises the bar for physicians to practice twenty-first century medicine and make the cultural switch from reactive medicine to evidenced-based healthcare. *"Evidence-based medicine is the conscientious, explicit, and judicious use of intelligence and knowledge in the care of individual patients. It is healthcare that combines a physician's best clinical expertise with credible external clinical evidence from systematic research."*[6]

Experienced clinicians typically use a wide range of judgments, decisions, actions, and recommendations in their practice of medicine. Their knowledge, past experience, respect for the patient's wishes, and an appreciation for the generally accepted practice rules within their community help them make decisions on care. Many healthcare institutions and professional associations have developed guidelines that are based on available evidence and expert opinion. Additionally, there are many databases available on the Internet that provide guidelines for various medical questions. For example, The American Society of Hematology and the American Board of Internal Medicine jointly developed a Web-based evaluation tool to assist physicians who treat a particular blood disorder called idiopathic thrombocytopenic purpura (ITP), characterized by easy bruising and excessive bleeding. This Web-based performance evaluation tool is the first nonmalignant hematology practice improvement module and provides an invaluable resource to physicians who treat patients with ITP. It is the availability and use of such Web-based technology that enables physicians to incorporate evidence-based clinical analysis into their decisions, along with relevant research, from the basic sciences; clinical examination of the patient, results of diagnostic tests, prognostic markers, and evaluations of the efficacy and safety of therapeutic, rehabilitative, and preventive approaches.

Evidence-based medical practice puts a great deal of responsibility on the individual clinician to stay abreast of and informed about advances using the available literature, online databases, and by attending symposia and meetings. It requires institutions that support physicians to provide the resources, leadership, vision, infrastructure, and an environment that fosters collaboration among various disciplines and specialties. From the many disparate data sources in the hospital or clinic, clinicians have the added burden of sorting, analyzing, and organizing the data into manageable sets of credible information that can be applied to patient care. There are many Web resources to assist in this process - that help elevate quality in medical practice. Incorporating these tools is not easy for the already overworked physician.[7]

Quality Initiatives Require Change

Building a quality clinical practice involves both innovation and change. However, change does not come easily to healthcare professionals who are tradition bound. Because of their labor intensive schedules, clinicians have little time for reflection and innovation. Twentieth century medical school training did not foster the idea of interactive digital communication with patients and use of extensive databases and online resources now available to the twenty-first century ehealth professional. Compounding the problem is the fact that today's patients expect more from a doctor than science and skill. They also evaluate their physicians based on the clinician's approach during the physical examination, the doctor's ability to provide health education, discussion of treatment options, consistency, elements of personal warmth and compassion, and the physician's communications ability. Sometimes the quality that is lacking in a particular clinician's care is not directly attributable to the physician but to how an office is run.

An elderly patient experiences two episodes of rectal bleeding and calls her physician's office twice in three hours. Both times she is put through to an answering machine. Several hours later she calls again and finally reaches a receptionist. She asks when it might be a good time to reach her physician by phone. She is put off by a "there is no good time response." The next morning the patient calls to request a visit with the doctor. She is told to call back the answering machine and leave a message because the doctor's secretary is on vacation. She calls the machine where she listens to a message that says she has to wait at least two weeks before she can be seen. Irate, concerned, stressed, this patient has no satisfactory recourse. She cannot seem to get the attention of the doctor and must either wait the two weeks or go to the emergency room at the local hospital. What is wrong with this picture?[8]

An answering machine in a practice should be used for urgent messages during off hours. Those messages should be transmitted to the healthcare professional as quickly as possible. A designated office associate should respond in a timely fashion to the patient. Although this does not quite represent the 24/7 availability of the IOM standards of care, patients are generally satisfied knowing that their clinician responds to their requests or question and respects their need for assistance so that they are not forced to go to the emergency room. In a healthcare crisis, patients want to know that their physician will take care of them at that time when they feel helpless and vulnerable.

Many industries have gone through extensive change to survive and maintain quality – some more successfully than others. For example, following deregulation in 1978, quality service became essential to the airline industry. During that period many airlines were forced to declare bankruptcy, and the survivors realized that they had to make changes to the way they were conducting their business. So they tried to reverse their priorities from focusing on profit to focusing on customer service. They worked to build a sense of pride and professionalism among their employees by shifting management policy away from punishing poor performance to a program of employee recognition that they hoped would motivate employees to improve performance. Although these quality initiatives became predominant, the airline industry has not been able to dig their way out of their state of chaos, which inhibits their ability to offer good customer service and make a profit at the same time.[9]

The automotive industry has also undergone sweeping change as automation hit the production line in the middle of the twentieth century. American auto companies were slow to admit to and adopt changes both in design and production as they faced heavy competition from the Japanese automakers that were producing better, faster, safer, cheaper automobiles. Toyota in particular had earned a reputation of high quality at low cost. From the start they established a value proposition that elevated quality control and quality standards that were sacred to their operation. With meticulous attention to meeting diverse customer preferences, they instituted systems that have enabled them to maintain just-in-time (JIT) production, which means they produce only what is needed and when it is needed. They also developed a process on the production line of identifying and correcting production problems when and where they happen. Their quality control engineers serve as an integral hands-on part of the team, always on the lookout to prevent problems from occurring.

The high technology companies that survived into the twenty-first century such as IBM, Intel, and Xerox also place strong emphasis on quality. They learned early on that the ability to think out of the box, act swiftly to sea changes in the marketplace, and elevate customer satisfaction to the top of their agenda would keep them viable.

Lessons Learned

The lessons learned from observing how these industries have fared in implementing change and quality initiatives point out the difficulties that healthcare organization will face as they elevate quality to the top of the agenda to better insure patient satisfaction and safer patient practices. Among the take away lessons are:

1. Effecting change is a collaborative process that begins with the reengineering of existing silos in an organization.
2. Establishing cross-functional teams that have the appropriate resources, education, and understanding of what makes the organization tick is critical to this process.
3. Vision and ideas are not enough. The organization needs to be pulled apart and realigned.
4. Adequate funding and resources are essential to achieving quality. Anything less results in a fragmented, partial solution.
5. Incentives and rewards that motivate people to change must be part of the overall plan to get everyone to buy into the process from the top down and the bottom up.
6. In healthcare, change must be focused on improving patient care. Patient feedback must be solicited via email campaigns and using exit interviews and online surveys when patients are released from the hospital or leaving the clinic.
7. Data are essential to the process of change. Full disclosure is the only way that change agents in an organization accomplish what they need to get done.
8. Nothing happens without commitment and support from the executive suite.

Resources

There are several nonprofit public policy organizations whose mission is to drive improvement in the quality, safety, and efficiency of healthcare through information and information technology. These organizations that bring together a wide range of stakeholders including clinicians, IT suppliers, health plans, healthcare purchasers, employers, hospitals, laboratories, patient and consumer groups, pharmaceutical and medical device manufacturers, public health agencies, representatives of state, regional, and community-based health organizations and employers. Physicians should be aware of the work of these organizations including:

The EHealth Initiative

The eHealth Initiative's focus is on educating policy makers and healthcare decision-makers about how the rapid adoption of interoperable information technology will advance clinical care, promote economic efficiencies, facilitate the linkage of a fragmented system, and give consumers the information they need to more effectively navigate the healthcare system. They promote the adoption of standards and advocate for laws, regulations, and policies that support technology and drive safety, quality, and efficiency throughout healthcare.
www.ehealthinitiative.org

Bridges to Excellence

The Bridges to Excellence programs are designed to provide incentives that reward physicians and practices for adopting better systems of care that result in physician practice reengineering, the adoption of health information technology, and delivering good outcomes to patients. Bridges to Excellence is a not-for-profit organization of employers, physicians, health care services, researchers, and other industry experts. Their mission is to promote quality of care by recognizing and rewarding health care providers who demonstrate that they have implemented comprehensive solutions in the management of patients and delivery of safe, timely, effective, efficient, equitable and patient-centered care.

Bridges to Excellence provides incentives for physicians that encourage them to focus on reengineering and ultimately improving their practice. Their Programs, funded by member organizations, include:

Physician Office Link (POL)

This enables physician office sites to qualify for bonuses based on their implementation of specific processes intended to reduce errors and increase quality. A report card for each physician office in the Bridges for Excellence program describes its performance on the program measures and is made available to the public.

Diabetes Care Link (DCL)

This enables physicians to achieve one-year or three-year recognition for high performance in diabetes care.

Cardiac Care Link (CCL)

This enables physicians to achieve three-year recognition for high performance in cardiac care.

Spine Care Link (SCL)

This enables physicians to achieve two-year recognition for high performance in spine care.

Each of these programs offer a suite of products and tools to help patients get engaged in their care, achieve better outcomes, and identify local physicians who meet high performance measures (http://www.bridgestoexcellence.org).

The Leapfrog Group

This organization works on behalf of the millions of Americans for whom many of the nation's largest corporations and public agencies buy health benefits, The Leapfrog Group provides reliable, meaningful information on hospital performance, enabling consumers and purchasers to compare the quality of care across hospitals that voluntarily participate in Leapfrog's two public reporting initiatives on hospital performance: Their goal is to reduce preventable medical mistakes. The Leapfrog Group has set up hospital safe practice criteria consisting of 27 procedures to reduce preventable medical error. They focus on proven practices in the hospital that have reduced unnecessary deaths, including the implementation of CPOE, and staffing the ICU with intensivists who have the training to treat the critically ill. Leapfrog's hallmark public reporting initiative has been a significant catalyst in advancing transparency of hospital performance (http://www.leapfroggroup.org).

The National Committee for Quality Assurance (NCQA)

The National Committee for Quality Assurance is a private, 501(c)(3) not-for-profit organization, that, since its founding in 1990, has been a central figure in driving quality improvement. The NCQA seal is a widely recognized symbol of quality.

Organizations incorporating the seal into advertising and marketing materials must first pass a rigorous, comprehensive review, and must annually report on their performance. NCQA's programs and services reflect a straightforward formula for improvement: *Measure. Analyze. Improve. Repeat.* NCQA makes this process possible in healthcare by developing quality standards and performance measures for a broad range of healthcare entities. These measures and standards are the tools that organizations and individuals can use to identify opportunities for improvement. The annual reporting of performance against such measures has become a focal point for the media, consumers, and health plans, which use these results to set their improvement agendas (http://www.ncqa.org).

Joint Commission on Accreditation of Healthcare Organizations' (JCAHO)

The JCAHO is an independent, not-for-profit organization that accredits and certifies more than 15,000 health care organizations and programs in the United States. Their accreditation and certification is recognized nationwide as a symbol of quality that reflects an organization's commitment to meeting certain performance standards. JCAHO's mission is to continuously improve the safety and quality of care provided to the public through the provision of health care accreditation and related services that support performance improvement in health care organizations. These services include the following:

* Accreditation
* Performance measurement
* Patient safety
* Information dissemination
* Public policy initiatives

The institutions that JCAHO surveys include clinical laboratories, critical access hospitals and a broad spectrum of disease specific care, and other certification programs. To earn and maintain the Joint Commission's Gold Seal of Approval, an organization must undergo an on-site survey at least every three years. (Laboratories must be surveyed every two years.) The purposes of the Joint Commission are backed and driven by the health care professional community – physicians, health care executives, nurses, pharmacists, and others. The beneficiaries of their work are the public. (http://www.jointcommission.org)

The Agency for Healthcare Research and Quality (AHRQ)

AHRQ, established in 1989 within the Department of Health and Human Services (HHS), is the lead Federal agency for researching and addressing healthcare costs, quality, outcomes, and patient safety by supporting research designed to identify the most effective ways to organize, manage, finance, and deliver high quality care, reduce medical errors and improve patient safety, particularly by using computers and other information technology in patient care.

Among their priorities are:

- Support for researchers and research networks that address concerns of very high public priority, such as health disparities, drugs and other therapeutics, primary care practice, and integrated health care delivery systems.
- Support for projects that test and evaluate successful methods that translate research into practice to improve patient care in diverse health care settings.
- Support for Evidence-based Practice Centers that review and synthesize scientific evidence for conditions or technologies that are costly, common, or important to the Medicare or Medicaid programs.
- Translation of the recommendations of the US Preventive Services Task Force into resources for providers, patients, and health care systems.

The AHRQ also oversees the operations of the Patient Safety Task Force, a Federal initiative designed to integrate research, data collection, and analysis of medical errors and promote interagency collaboration in reducing the number of injuries resulting from these errors. They provide hospitals, health data organizations, and States with enhanced quality assessment tools that they can use with their own hospital administrative data to highlight potential quality concerns and track changes over time in three areas: ambulatory care sensitive conditions, inpatient quality (volume, mortality, and resource use), and patient safety (http://www.ahrq.gov).

The Malcolm Baldrige National Quality Award

The Malcolm Baldrige National Quality Award was created by Public Law 100–107, signed into law on August 20, 1987. Initially targeted to American industry to recognize companies that were working toward improving the quality of the goods and services they provide, the Malcolm Baldrige award established new standards of excellence based upon a rigorous set of requirements that included a wide range of quality measurements that had to be in place over a period of time.

Originally three types of organizations were eligible for the Baldrige awards: manufacturers, service companies, and small businesses. This was expanded in 1999 to include education and healthcare institutions; again in 2007 to include nonprofit organizations, including trade and professional organizations charities and government agencies.

The Baldridge awards for healthcare set out requirements for performance excellence in seven categories:

1. Leadership
2. Strategic planning
3. Focus on patients, other customers, and markets

4. Measurement, analysis, and knowledge management
5. Workforce focus
6. Process management
7. Results

In 2007, Mercy Health System in Janesville Wisconsin and Sharp Healthcare in San Diego CA were recipients of Baldrige National Quality Awards (http://www.quality. nist.gov).

Centers for Medicare and Medicaid Services (CMS)

Because increasing numbers of aging Americans get their healthcare coverage from the Centers for Medicare and Medicaid Services (CMS), their role in adopting and fostering quality in healthcare is closely followed and has an impact on the health-care industry as a whole. Since 2002, CMS has supported collaborative quality initiatives in nursing home, home health, and hospital settings, with a focus on making publicly available measures of provider performance on quality measures on its *"Compare Website."* More recently, the Agency has begun to link these meas-ures to provider reimbursement, with payment related to reporting of quality data, and ultimately to performance on these measures. http://www.cms.hhs.gov/ HospitalQualityInits/11_HospitalCompare.asp

In July 2005, CMS published the Quality Improvement Roadmap, a structured Quality Improvement Organization (QIO) Program consisting of a national network of 53 QIOs, responsible for each US state, territory, and the District of Columbia. QIOs work with consumers and physicians, hospitals, and other caregivers to refine care delivery systems to make sure patients get the right care at the right time, particularly patients from underserved populations. Over the past decade, the QIO Program has been an important national resource. Through its Website, http://www.medqic.org, the Program offers comprehensive information and tools related to best practices and ideas for change on a variety of topics in nursing home, home health, hospital, and physician office settings.

In 2007, CMS also created the hospital quality overview, a Website where con-sumers can find information on quality practices in a hospital, including:

- Data that indicate how often a hospital provides appropriate treatment for heart attacks, heart failure, pneumonia, surgery.
- A checklist for patients to review before choosing a particular hospital that includes such issues as whether or not the hospital has experience and is accred-ited for treating a particular condition; whether or not it is flexible in allowing families to participate and support a patient's care, and whether or not the hos-pital has an appropriate level of cleanliness.

CMS has taken a leadership role on Personal Health Records, and encourages its beneficiaries to establish a PHR at the CMS portal, http://www.mymedicare.gov.

They have also mandated that physicians move to eprescribing technology (http://www.cms.hhs.gov).

We are at the threshold of the ability of our information tools to deliver the best medical knowledge to the point of care, just in time. For years medical guidelines have decayed in textbooks and journals never to be applied when they were most needed. Many of these guidelines were promulgated without the bright light of clinical application, which would refine the best and eliminate the rest. In an era of the disappearance of the family doctor and ascension of the healthcare bank account, we more than ever need the routine reliable effective introduction of the best medical knowledge applied to our care before it is too late. Our healthcare information infrastructure is the only instrument that can deliver on that goal. It will not have achieved this potential a moment too soon.

Key Points

1. Quality is an initiative involving every member of the healthcare industry and it takes change on the part of every individual, group, and department to achieve the Institute of Medicine's Standards of Care.
2. Implementation of digital communication technology is an integral piece of the quality solution.
3. The patient is at the center of care and must be included in the change process and be thought of as the central focus of healthcare. Quality care is safe care for every patient, at every occurrence.
4. Quality care also is respectful of the individual patient's gender, background, ethnicity, geography, and socioeconomic status. None of this should make a difference in the approach to care in spite of the issue of insured vs. uninsured.
5. Evidenced-based medicine uses information resources to bring depth and broad understanding to a wide variety of issues that may not have been taught in medical school but are critical to making the right decision for the twenty-first century patient.
6. Patients have far more information at their fingertips than they can deal with and the healthcare professional practicing safe medicine must provide appropriate guidelines and filters to help patients use this plethora of information appropriately.
7. Every patient who seeks the advice of a physician truly believes that their healthcare issue is the only one on the physician's radar screen. They expect to receive full attention, quick response, and respect from their healthcare provider. All of these elements are part of quality care.
8. Physicians must use information resources to remain current so they bring to their practice a depth and broad understanding of many issues that may not have been taught in Medical School.

9. Part of the context for health decisions comes from external factors. Long waits, growing frustration, loss of control all destroy the quality of the patient's experience and can lead to unsafe practice. The physician needs to be aware of these external factors.

10. The physician must become a change agent, implementing twenty-first century digital tools: the Internet, email, PDAs, eprescribing, and applying evidence-based medicine to meet the stringent requirements expected of an eHealth professional.

11. Healthcare in the twenty-first century is a partnership between healthcare professionals and patients. The professionals need to help patient to empower themselves, using digital communication tools to understand fully what is going on and to participate fully with complete information to make decisions about their health.

References and Notes

1. www.photius.com/rankings/healthrank.htm
2. *Crossing the Quality Chasm, "Health care Today Harms Too Frequently and routinely fails to deliver its potential benefits", Donlan et al 1999 Reed St. Peter 1997; Shindul-Rothschild et al 1996; Taylor 2001*
3. *Crossing The Quality Chasm p. 5,6*
4. *Crossing the Quality Chasm, p. 8, 9*
5. *Health Information Technology for Improving Quality of Care in Primary Care Settings Agency for Healthcare Research and Quality* Prepared by Jerry Langley and Carol Beasley Institute for Healthcare Improvement July 2007 www.ihi.org/IHI/topics/improvement.htm
6. Sackett, D.L. et al. 13 January (1996) Evidence based medicine: what it is and what it isn't. BMJ 312 (7023), 71–72 (This paper is available on the Web at: http://cebm.jr2.ox.ac.uk/ebmisisnt.html)
7. The Promises and Pitfalls of Evidence-Based Medicine   **Stefan Timmermans and Aaron Mauck** Health Affairs, 24, no. 1 (2005): 18–28 doi: 10.1377/hlthaff.24.1.18 © 2005 by Project HOPE Science Daily Mar 20 2007, Online Tool Helps Physicians Improve Care of Patients with Bleeding Disorder www.sciencedaily.com/releases2007/03/070319180048.htm
8. Massachusetts Medical Society "Patient Satisfaction" 2004 www.massmed.org/cme
9. Harvard Business School cases: 9-491-036: Northwest Airlines Confronts Changes and 9-491-061 American Airlines: (C) Committing to Leadership

Chapter 10
Heathcare 2020

Baby James is born on February 12, 2020 at 3 am. Minutes after his birth, a micro-chip, the size of a grain of rice, is embedded in his arm. That microchip points to a Web site that was created within 24 hours of James's birth. It is coded with an assigned number that will belong to James for the rest of his life, no matter where in the world he may go. At this site all of the tests James was given: the PKU, the APGA, James's blood type and DNA, genetic markers analysis of James stem cells, and skin tissue, immunizations, results from a hearing test, a thumb print, and a scan of his retina, his birth certificate and other important information will be stored forever. James (or his family until he becomes of age) will own and control access to this record, which will be available in digital format. It will be available on a need-to-know basis to health care providers to whom the family or James has given consent. This immediate access to James's information eliminates the need for duplicate tests or interventions. It provides the right information for James at the point of care no matter where or when he needs healthcare services.

A Portrait

This is healthcare 2020 where critical clinical information is available, always, in an accurate, comprehensive format; where all patients are health literate because from birth, health is an important aspect of their lives; where 24/7 contact with a doctor via a virtual meeting on a television or computer screen or on a PDA or face-to-face in the clinic is possible. As wireless networks and handheld devices untether individuals from their desktops, communication between patient and an eHealth professional happen wherever those individuals happen to be–in the car, at the beach, watching a movie. Individuals can proactively send the doctor vitals, images, questions, and descriptions that are analyzed and feedback is immediate. Healthcare 2020 changes the healthcare dynamic from episodic encounters between physicians and their patients to a continuous care model where providers have full access to healthcare data on every patient when and where the patient needs it, because that microchip planted at birth points to the encrypted data at all times.

N.B. Finn and W.F. Bria, *Digital Communication in Medical Practice*,
DOI: 10.1007/978-1-84882-355-6_11, © Springer-Verlag London Limited 2009

Physicians and technicians perform routine tests and examinations in the patient's home or office via connected EKGs, EEGs, portable telehealth units that include tactile devices in the form of hats, gloves, floor mats, bracelets, and toothbrushes. The handheld cell phone, PDA, and MP3 player are in one device that enables this close communication.

The embedded microchip that every person now has lasts indefinitely. It transmits a unique 15-digit number that can be read by a handheld scanner that every healthcare organization keeps available. The microchip points to an electronic health record. There is no longer a question of who owns, pays for, and maintains the health record. In Healthcare 2020, the electronic health record is owned by the individual and accessed and updated by eHealth professionals, as appropriate, with permission of the patient. The record sits in a large data repository where maximum security standards are mandated by legislation and maintained. Bandwidth is no longer an issue. Digital networks use cable, fiber optics, and satellite communications for the access channels to carry out these interactions with ease. The infrastructure to support so many virtual health encounters has been built by an alliance of government agencies, community health agencies, health professionals, public health consortiums, hospitals, individuals, employers, educators, insurers, and patients. The goal of attaining interoperable health information technology that promotes quality, efficiency, and patient safety has been met. Highly specialized metropolitan care centers are in place for complex health services; walk in clinics exist for routine matters. Access to healthcare is everywhere and there are policies in place that make it available to everyone.

The overall cost of healthcare in 2020 continues to rise due to the increasing numbers of aging citizens and their demands on the system. The World Healthcare Organization predicts that by 2020 the population of over 65 individual's approaches 16.8 million with an estimated 90% of people living in their own home with healthcare support they need made available to them. There are 20.5 million people who suffer from long-term conditions. There is also much research that shows that even as far back as the middle of the twentieth century, during the last 60 days of life there is a disproportionate amount of money spent on healthcare that impacts on resources available throughout the system.[1]

A coalition of government, private organizations, employers, hospitals, physicians, payers, and foundations now oversee how we pay for care, who pays, and how we overcome the inequities in the system. A series of tax incentives and legislated regulations mandates that 2020 employers, large and small, provide all employees with basic healthcare during their work tenure and for up to 18 months after they cease to work as an employee, unless they opt out. Small companies that cannot afford this coverage are assisted through Federal programs and quasi-public agencies set up for this purpose. Individual's extraordinary health expenses come out of the health accounts that they set up either with matching grants from their employers or with personal funds, depending upon their income level. Those who cannot afford health accounts, who are unemployed, disabled, or otherwise unable to work, are supported by public funds. The increased use of digital technology including Web-based provider interactions, extensive deployment of telemedicine, remote surgeries via robots and other devices, and decision support systems help to control costs and elevate the quality of care that every person receives. Artificial intelligence in medical devices and systems including digital machines provide the solutions to previously unsolvable issues.

Patients in 2020 are offered incentives and the education that keeps them on track regarding health issues. In addition to the fact that they have mobile devices to help them stay in close communication with their eHealth professionals, they also are more thoroughly briefed in how diet, blood pressure, blood sugar, cholesterol, and other critical markers that indicate good health, should be kept in check. Individuals who follow the good health recommendations including losing weight, stopping smoking, controlling blood pressure are rewarded with funds contributed to their health accounts through a quasi-public foundation set up for this purpose. This is part of the high value that is placed on healthy living. It is not easy to make the system equitable for everyone but a process is in place that attempts to provide universal coverage for basic healthcare and legislated, care evaluation procedures when extraordinary situations arise that present a drain on the system for everyone including determinations on how to appropriately handle care for terminally ill patients.

Patients are also encouraged to interact with other individuals who have similar health problems through an abundance of online communities where assistance, support, and encouragement are available. These online communities have become part of the culture and provide a group dynamic that is especially helpful to individuals suffering from chronic diseases or other unusual problems and need the empathy, encouragement, and contact with others.

In Healthcare 2020, communication among systems is as transparent as telephone or email communications was in 2010. Systems made by one particular vendor easily transfer a communication–a call, video, or digital data to a system made by a different vendor because the standards and protocols to support a common interface are in place to bridge previous gaps in health information exchange. This easy transfer of information promotes better communication among physicians and other healthcare professionals and between healthcare professionals and their patients.

Privacy issues still loom large on the Healthcare 2020 horizon, dark and threatening. The more digital data we have, the more there is to be penetrated, and although the points of entry are more tightly controlled with advanced encryption technology and scanning capabilities (retinal scanning of individuals before accessing a record), there is always an underlying threat. Human nature being what it is, patients in 2020 have reason to fear that with sophisticated digital records, savvy individuals or companies who desire to access those records for profit or illicit purposes can and will do so.

By 2020 every Medical School has incorporated health information technol-ogy into their curriculum so that graduating physicians have undergone training in the value and the logistics of electronic health records, telemedicine, Internet resources, CPOE, privacy issues, and business questions related to HIT. This change in their training produces physicians who are more entrepreneurial and open to a constantly changing healthcare landscape promulgating more rapid adoption of new technology.

Devices and Enablers

There are a number of devices that were developed in the first decade of the twenty-first century that have made Healthcare 2020 possible:

Personal Digital Assistants and Smart Phones

PDAs started out as calendars and address books then memos were added and email, Internet access, cameras, and GPS devices that can actually pinpoint a patient's exact location. By 2020, these PDAs are able to transmit a patient's blood pressure, heart rate, and other vital signs, as well as a graphic image of an individual or a specific part of the body that requires examination. These same PDAs provide physicians with access to drug information and intelligent decision support tools for immediate accurate diagnostic assistance. Cellular telephones preceded the PDAs. They began life as simple wireless telephones. Email and access to the Internet were added to the cell phone, along with instant/text messaging, cameras, and MP3 players. In the early part of the twenty-first century, cell phones and PDAs were integrated into a single device that even contains chips that enable the device to be used as a debit card as well as a communication tool. The molecular wireless device of Healthcare 2020 includes unique applications including DNA chips capable of analyzing molecules from an individual's body to alert the individual about a virus, infection, or a sudden rise or drop in blood pressure, blood sugar, or oxygen level. The potential is limitless as the PDA or smart phone evolves into a diagnostic device that benefits the individual and the physician.

Radio Frequency Identification (RFID)

Radio frequency identification (RFID) is a technology where tiny transmitters, embedded in a tag or bracelet, send out an encoded stream of bits to alert a reader. During the first decade of the century, RFID technology was used to match an identifier on a patient with an identifier on a pill container or other medication container to check that the right patient is given the right drug at the right dosage. RFID has also been used to track materials, medications, and patients in the hospital to reduce medical error and promote patient safety. This includes specimen collection, blood administration, and medication administration, nursing workflow and tracking processes, patient movement as well as tracking medical equipment throughout the hospital.

In Healthcare 2020 with RFID technology, efficiency and economies of scale are in place so that healthcare institutions no longer experience huge costs to replace instruments that have been lost or misplaced, or to locate drugs that are missing, or to find patients kept waiting in the surgical centers and in the ER, or to track blood supplies and transfusion packets that need to be administered correctly to the right individuals. RFID enables physicians to read the microchips that point them to databases for critical information on patients or help them find informational data on the Internet that they need.

Robots

Robots are mechanical devices that, through built-in microprocessors and sensors, are capable of performing a variety of complex human tasks on command or by being programmed in advance. They typically operate via remote control. Robots used in healthcare are equipped with a set of medical sensors enabling them to measure blood pressure, heart rate, heartbeat irregularities, and body temperature. They perform a number of functions that help in the care of the elderly or chronically ill patients, for example: addressing cognitive decline by reminding patients to drink, to take medicine, or helping them to remember an appointment. They are also used for collecting data, monitoring for emergencies such as heart failure, and assisting people with domestic tasks.

By the beginning of the twenty-first century robots capable of performing complex assignments were developed to assist human surgeons in performing minimally invasive surgery. Since their precision is extremely accurate, they reduce the number of people needed in the operating room during procedures and enhance surgical performance with their superior dexterity. In 2020, robots are found everywhere providing expertise coverage that is cost effective and handling surgical tasks too difficult for the human hand. Robotic tele-rounding is common practice. A six-foot tall robot equipped with a 15-inch flat screen, two high-resolution cameras, and a microphone enables two-way video conferencing as it makes rounds and sees patients. A live conversation and visit between a patient and a doctor, who remotely controls the robot through an Internet connection, takes place. The physician appears on the screen and carries on a conversation with the patient as easily as if he or she were physically present. The doctor remotely drives the robot through the hospital to each patient's room to check patient's vital signs, inspect incisions, and discuss treatment options in real time. Specialists who may be hundreds of miles away also use robots to virtually consult with patients. There are robots that help in the emergency room by connecting a patient with a distant specialist and other robots that monitor patients in the intensive care unit working with a physician who is sitting in a remote location. This takes the eICU to another level where the physician can observe, examine, and interact with the patient extending the physician's ability to be available at the patient's bedside 24/7.

Telemedicine

Telemedicine networks are everywhere in 2020. They are in the large urban centers where they provide home monitoring services to the elderly and the home-bound patients who cannot get to the doctor or the hospital for care. They are in remote areas where distances prevents many citizens from getting the medical care they need for both standard care and in a crisis. A cadre of individuals including: primary care physicians, nurse practitioners, nurses, and specialists are available through special care telemedicine units that are located throughout the country. State legislation no longer prevents physicians from practicing medicine across state lines. Those regulations were abolished long ago to enable specialists from major medical centers to be available as needed to individuals wherever they may be. The combination of RFID technology and robotics enables telemedicine in 2020 to insure skilled care for everyone.

Decision Support and Evidenced-Based Medicine

Intelligent decision support systems of 2020 put patient information at the center of healthcare. Vast data repositories containing comprehensive records on millions of patients allow the physician to enter a query that includes patient characteristics such as age, weight, gender, and preexisting conditions. Electronic information from multiple data sources using data mining tools returns unbiased, evidence-based guidance that results in high quality treatment options based on proven patterns and usage. These same databases return user information to help patients understand their treatment choices and collaborate effectively with their doctors. Additionally, the accumulated knowledge resident in the data repository about the genetic roots of many chronic diseases such as asthma, various cancers, diabetes, heart disease along with the PHR that includes a patient's DNA enables physicians to get fast, accurate analyses. Patient privacy is protected because within these data repositories patient identities are kept separate from research data. Real-time clinical surveillance tools scan the available data for preset triggers that warn of adverse drug events to avoid medical or medication errors from occurring.

Surgery

Surgery in 2020 is also driven by intuitive communications and sensor technologies that support highly trained and cohesive teams who get the patient in and out of surgery as quickly and effectively as possible. Once the decision is made for surgery, expert software examines the patient's medical history, as well as aggregate and surgeon-specific outcomes experience for a contemplated procedure. Presurgical testing, diagnostic studies, and interventions driven by the software analysis are chosen. A secure Website specific to this case is launched where appointments are coordinated and test results are disseminated to appropriate stakeholders, including doctors, nurses, and the patient who is also able to review, online, the educational material tailored for the specific procedure. Specific reminders, perioperative instructions, and information are posted for the patient. Meanwhile automated supply management dispenses RFID tagged supplies for the scheduled surgery based on a moving window of the surgeon's past use of items for the booked procedure. In areas where surgery is needed but the specialists are not available to perform the procedures, robots, which are controlled remotely by distant specialists, stand in and perform the procedure. The local doctor, nurse practitioner, or nurses stand by ready to assist where needed.

Personalized Medicine

On October 27, 2005, The International HapMap consortium published a comprehensive catalog of more than 1 million human genetic variations grouped in blocks called haplotypes. This HapMap database allows researchers to compare the genetic sequences of different individuals to identify chromosomal regions where genetic variants are shared. This is the essence of personalized medicine, where a doctor can test a patient's DNA and check for variations that cause adverse reactions to a broad range of drugs and treatments. By comparing people who have the same disease, such as diabetes, and by comparing individual responses to therapeutic agents, researchers are able to find common markers (haplotypes) (http://hapmap.org/healthbenefit.html.en).

These discoveries enable healthcare professionals in 2020 to know much more about the origins of illnesses and about ways to prevent, diagnose, and treat illness. For example, knowing how each person's body handles different drugs, physicians are able to prescribe the right amount of the right drug rather than having to guess. Some people are slow to metabolize Dilantin, while others will metabolize it rapidly. A genetic test can identify how the drug will process in an individual. As of 2008, genetic tests were available clinically for more than 900 diseases. Genetic testing has evolved from a pursuit primarily of academic laboratories studying rare diseases, to a technology that has become part of mainstream medicine and encompasses a wide net that includes predispositional testing and accurate diagnostic assessments that result in new treatments and responses.[2]

By 2020, DNA sequencing research is at a point where treatments are customized based on a patient's genetic make-up, to maximize effectiveness and minimize side effects. Genetic variants contributing to longevity or resistance to disease provide the pathway for new therapies with widespread benefits. A patient who knows their personal risk for a particular disease makes the appropriate lifestyle changes and engages in more aggressive disease surveillance and preventive medical treatments. This personalized information-based health care, which rests on scientific information and not conjecture, has transformed medicine, enabling the physician to know what works, why it works, and who it works for resulting in patient care that is easily customized and optimized for each individual.

Virtual Reality

Virtual reality (VR) is a human-computer interface that simulates a realistic environment and allows users to interact with it. Most current VR programs are visual experiences, displayed either on a computer screen or through special stereoscopic displays. These simulations include sensory information, through speakers or headphones. Advanced, sensory systems used in medicine may include tactile information. VR emerged as an accepted scientific discipline for medicine in the first decade of the twenty-first century. The majority of VR applications have been in the area of surgery, although use in rehabilitative medicine and psychiatry has also been significant. Virtual endoscopy, which may replace standard endoscopic procedures for diagnostic screening is also emerging. The most highly developed area of VR is in surgical simulations. The types of simulations range from needle-based procedures, such as standard intravenous insertion, central venous placement catheter, and chest-tube insertion to more sophisticated simulations of full surgical procedures like laparoscopic cholecystectomy. In addition, haptic input devices are providing the sense of touch to the procedures.

By 2020 much of a surgeon's training encompasses VR. Additionally, patient-specific models derived from computed tomography or magnetic resonance imaging scans that permit surgeons and neurosurgeons to practice a delicate surgical procedure on the patient's specific virtual anatomy before actually performing the procedure on the patient. These applications afford the surgeon the opportunity to provide the highest surgical care possible through the use of advanced technologies. Other uses of VR include the following:

Binge-eating: By interacting with food in a virtual world, patients learn to control appetite
Pain: VR that distract adults and children when they are undergoing minor surgery
Stroke: VR to retrain the brains of stroke victims
Burns: VR that can help to ease burn victims' pain

Diagnosing disease based on a patient's DNA profile, blood sample, and a CT body scan that looks at the entire body and produces a simulated digital reproduction enables the physician in 2020 to confront complex medical problems and the mysteries of disease and pinpoint the exact cause, location, and actions that the patient needs with confidence.

The Practice of Medicine in Healthcare 2020

The cornerstone of healthcare practice in 2020 is that the patient occupies center stage, not the physician. With the digital personal health record that is owned and always available to an empowered patient and easily accessible to every healthcare professional as needed, interactions take place whenever and wherever feasible via face to face visits, house calls, on a Web portal, in a quick response clinic or in the traditional doctor's office or the hospital emergency room. All of the fundamental healthcare services are provided to individuals by a healthcare gatekeeper, who is responsible for coordinating care, controlling costs, and communicating results to the patient. Providers also work with the healthcare community to insure that the best resources are available. Advances in telecommunications, medical imaging, massive intelligent databases memory miniaturization, satellite technology, and other information systems allows physicians to communicate far more easily and quickly, and enables patients to educate and empower themselves to take responsibility for their health.

Patients are served in a number of ways. Those who live in urban and suburban centers and who are too elderly or infirm to leave their place of residence are visited at least quarterly by a core of physicians, who along with their nurses and nurse practitioners make house calls. These same patients are monitored daily at the telemedicine centers. Face time with the physician is supplemented with Web visits. This approach prevents an illness from getting out of control resulting in a critical care emergency landing in the ER. With portable computing technology and robot assistants, this approach works well and provides assistance and comfort for the lonely and often depressed homebound individuals.

For mobile patients, there are a number of outlets for accessing healthcare. Retail clinics, which became a factor early in the twenty-first century, are spread across the country and are available to everyone to address the routine problems. According to a Forrester Research Inc. survey (see Figure 10.1) conducted in 2006, convenient schedules and locations drive consumers to retail clinics. Unlike most doctors' offices, retail clinics are often open weekends and nights and promise to treat consumers within 15 min with no appointments necessary. Treatment is generally with a nurse or nurse practitioner and more serious cases are sent to the local hospital. Nearly a quarter of individuals surveyed felt that clinics offer the same level of quality that is offered by other health delivery options.

In Healthcare 2020, people routinely use retail clinics for issues that are not complex but need immediate attention such as colds and coughs, ear aches, cuts and bruises, stomach complaints, flu-related symptoms and strep throat. These clinics are located at the neighborhood pharmacy, in large retail centers, strip malls, and business centers. Many of the clinics have a loose affiliation with a local hospital. They are subject to oversight by governmental health agencies to see that they maintain a level of quality and safety in their practice. Health insurers happily pay for these visits that are much less costly than a trip to the ER.

The task of managing the resources of healing is one of the most complex and difficult enterprises on the planet. Healthcare 2020 optimizes the care model with a team of eHealth professionals who use technology to provide the best available care to patients. The focus in primary care is both prevention and chronic disease coordination. The 2020 eHealth professional's role and responsibility has changed from one of intervening in acute disease, to early screening, detection, treatment, and prevention, which controls expenses. It is an uphill battle to provide quality healthcare to everyone, but is a battle that must be won if all the citizens of the earth are to survive and thrive.

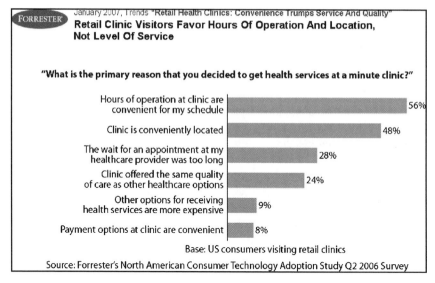

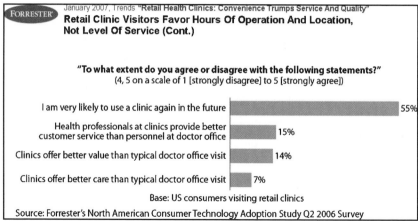

Figure 10.1 Retail clinic visitors favor hours of operation and location, not level of service

Key Points

1. The availability of information technology that fosters the potential for 24/7 communication between eHealth professionals and patients forms the essence of their relationship in Healthcare 2020.
2. A microchip embedded in every individual, which points to a personal health record residing on a secure site on the Internet, resolves the issue of who owns the record and how it is accessed by the many providers that an individual deals with.
3. Universal basic health coverage is the norm in 2020. Individuals have to plan for and save for extraordinary health expenses. Those who are not employed have

access to healthcare coverage through a collaborative of private and public funds.

4. Patients are educated, motivated, and incented to pay attention to their health and work toward a healthy life style, thus curbing their need for healthcare services.

5. Physicians are taught through medical school education and continuing education about the logistics and value of information technology. It becomes part of their everyday professional life.

6. Many devices and enablers including: smart PDAs, RFID, robots, universal telemedicine networks, decision support systems comprise the HIT environment and foster better, safer medicine for everyone.

7. Personalized Medicine, based on our understanding of the human genome, fosters healthcare that changes medicine in several ways including: more effective ways to predict individual susceptibility to disease; more useful and person-specific tools for preventing disease, greater ability to detect the onset of disease, based on makers and preempting the progression of disease.

8. VR simulations provide a mechanism for training physicians and enabling researchers to better understand the human body, raising the standards of care for many diseases, and conditions.

9. The patient has become the cornerstone of healthcare in 2020 and patients are served in many ways from home monitoring to retail clinics to Web visits to traditional care in the doctor's office or at the hospital.

References and Notes

1. www.e-health-insider.com/News/2441 August 4, 2008.
2. Personalized Medicine: The "Perfect Storm" for Improving Genetic Test Quality - By Kathy Hudson* and Gail Javitt** February 20, 2006 www.dnapolicy.org/resources

Glossary

These items are included to clarify the use of this terminology in this book. They should not be interpreted as approved terms or definitions but considered as contextual descriptions. Resources used in compiling this glossary include input from the National Alliance for Health Information Technology (NAHIT), a consortium of healthcare executives mandated to define commonly used health IT terms, and Wikipedia, the largest multilingual free online encyclopedia.

Adherence: Patients' following a prescribed treatment ordered by a physician including the taking of medications at the times dosages prescribed.

Adverse Event: A change in health or "side-effect" that occurs in a person during a clinical trial or other health-related circumstance. Adverse events may be related to drugs, vaccinations, devices, procedures, patient care, and other health events.

American Health Information Community (AHIC): A Federal advisory body chartered in 2005, serving to make recommendations to the Secretary of the US Department of Health and Human Services regarding the development and adoption of health information technology.

American National Standards Institute (ANSI) H.32x: A standard enabling video-conferencing and interoperability that has helped develop telemedicine technology allowing patients and providers to interact independent of the particular hardware in place.

American National Standards Institute (ANSI) Healthcare Information Technology Standards Panel (HITSP): A body created in 2005 to promote interoperability and harmonization of healthcare information technology through standards that enable cooperation among public and private sectors.

Certification Commission for Healthcare Information Technology (CCHIT): This organization is mandated to set criteria and help accelerate the adoption of health information technology.

Centers for Disease Control and Prevention (CDC): A Federal agency within the Department of Health and Human Services that serves to enhance and promote the health and quality of life by preventing and controlling disease, injury, and disability. Working with states and other partners, CDC provides a system of health surveillance to monitor and prevent disease outbreaks (including bioterrorism), implements disease prevention strategies, and maintains national health statistics. CDC also provides for immunization services, workplace safety, and environmental disease prevention. CDC also guards against international disease transmission.

Centers for Medicare & Medicaid Services (CMS): A Federal agency within the Department of Health and Human Services that administers Medicare, Medicaid, and the State Children's Health Insurance Program through portability standards.

Collaborative Drug Therapy: Collaboration between pharmacists and physicians to serve patient's medication needs.

Common Procedural Terminology (CPT): Reimbursement codes set by the American Medical Association that establishes fees for medical services and procedures.

Consumers: Members of the public including patients, caregivers, patient advocates, surrogates, family members, and other parties who may be acting for, or in support of, a patient receiving or potentially receiving healthcare services.

Consumer Driven Health Plans (CDHP): Health benefits plans that engage covered individuals in choosing their own health care providers, managing their own health expenses, and improving their own health with respect to factors that they can control.

Computer Physician Order Entry (CPOE): A computer-based system for writing orders in the hospital setting for medication and treatment that eliminates the need for transcription and improves medical documentation. CPOE software may be bundled with decision support software.

Decision Support: An activity that enables improved analysis and conclusions based on related information, recent research, algorithms, or other resources. In a clinical environment, decision support can help clinicians make more informed care decisions based on these resources. Clinical decision support is a related activity with specific components such as best practice guidelines, medication contraindication information, and access to recent research.

Digital Imaging and Communication in Medicine (DICOM): A standard for handling, storing, printing, and transmitting information in medical imaging. It includes a file format definition and a network communications protocol. The communication protocol is an application protocol that uses TCP/IP to communicate between systems. DICOM files can be exchanged between two entities that are capable of receiving image and patient data in DICOM format.

eHealth: The delivery of healthcare services that incorporates the use of information technology and fosters a collaborative environment between a patient and a provider that includes sharing of information and interactive communication.

eHealth Professionals: Those healthcare providers who have incorporated information technology into their practice.

eHospitals: Organizations that have implemented digital communication technology tools to admit track and treat patients.

eICU: A location that is removed from the physical Intensive Care Unit where a physician can monitor several ICUs at the same time. The eICU can be located within a hospital complex or off site miles away and is manned 24/7 by intensive care doctors and nurses.

Electronic Health Record (EHR): An aggregate electronic record of health-related information on an individual that conforms to nationally recognized interoperability standards and that can be created, managed, and consulted by authorized clinicians and staff across more than one health care organization. The EHR includes patient demographics, progress notes, problems, medications, medical history, immunizations, laboratory data, and radiology reports and images (source: NAHIT).

Electronic Mail: The sending of messages through the Internet

Electronic Medical Record: An electronic record of health-related information on an individual that can be created, gathered, managed, and consulted by authorized clinicians and staff within one health care organization (source: NAHIT).

Electronic Prescribing (e-prescribing): Entering a prescription into an automated data entry system and generating that prescription electronically.

ePatients: Those individuals who use available information technology including the Internet and email to interact with their healthcare providers and seek information on health issues.

eVisit: An asynchronous online discussion between a clinician and a patient via the Internet, in a secure environment.

Evidenced-Based Medicine: Practice of medicine that uses the best external resources available, including clinical evidence from research to make judgments and decisions about patient care.

Food and Drug Administration (FDA): US Federal Agency responsible for protecting the public health by assuring the safety, efficacy, and security of human and veterinary drugs, biological products, medical devices, food supply, cosmetics, and products that emit radiation.

Forrester Research Inc. An independent technology and market research company that focuses on technology's impact on business and industry.

Hapolotypes: Genetic variations grouped into blocks.

HapMap: Describes the common patterns of human DNA sequence variation. The HapMap database is a key resource for researchers to use to find genes affecting health, disease, and responses to drugs and environmental factors.

Healthcare Effectiveness Data and Information Set (HEDIS): A way of measuring delivery of healthcare on various dimensions of care and service to determine the P4P rate.

Health Information Exchange (HIE): The electronic movement of health-related data and information including email, the Internet, digital databases, audio and video, among organizations according to specific standards, protocols, and other agreed criteria (source: NAHIT).

Healthcare Information and Management Systems Society (HIMSS): A US not-for-profit organization dedicated to promoting a better understanding of health care information and management systems.

Health Information Technology (HIT): The deployment of digital communication tools including email, the Internet, digital databases, audio and video, to facilitate information exchange among healthcare providers and patients.

Health Insurance Portability Accountability Act (HIPAA): Legislation enacted in 1996 by the US Congress to protect health insurance coverage for workers and their families when they change or lose their job and to define national standards for electronic healthcare transactions and address the privacy and security of health data.

Health Level Seven (HL7): An all-volunteer, not-for-profit organization involved in development of international healthcare standards. "HL7" is also used to refer to some of the specific standards, which support clinical practice and the management, delivery, and evaluation of health services, that are the most commonly used in the world.

Health Maintenance Organization (HMO): An organization that provides health care coverage in the United States fulfilled through hospitals, doctors, and other providers with which the HMO has a contract. The HMO covers only care rendered by those doctors and other professionals who have agreed to treat patients in accordance with the HMO's guidelines and restrictions in exchange for a steady stream of patients.

Health Practice Shortage Area (HPSA): A region in the United States where there is a shortage of primary care physicians, dentists, and mental health practitioners as defined by CMS.

Healthcare Payers: Insurers, including health plans, self-insured employer plans, and third party administrators, providing healthcare benefits to enrolled members and reimbursing provider organizations.

Health Reimbursement Accounts (HRA): Funds that are set aside by an employer on behalf of an employee for healthcare needs.

Health Savings Accounts (HSA): Funds set up to assist individuals with payment of out of pocket health expenses; both employers and employees contribute to the HSA up to an annual amount limit set by statutory cap.

Institute of Medicine (IOM): One of the United States' National Academies, this is a not for profit nongovernmental organization whose purpose is to provide advice on a variety of issues related to biomedical science, medicine, and health. Each IOM report is reviewed by the expert panel that includes physician's scientists and others.

National Committee for Quality Assurance (NCQA): A private, 501(c)(3) not-for-profit organization dedicated to improving health care quality. Since its founding in 1990, NCQA has been a central figure in driving improvement in quality standards.

National E-Prescribing Patient Safety Initiative (NEPSI): A joint project of several healthcare organizations with the goal of providing free e-prescribing software to every physician in the United States to address medical error in the prescribing process.

NHS: The National Health Service of the United Kingdom.

ONC: Office of the National Coordinator for Health Information Technology; serves as the HHS Secretary's principal advisor on the development, application, and use of health information technology in an effort to improve the quality, safety, and efficiency of the nation's health through the development of an interoperable harmonized health information infrastructure.

Patient Portal: A secure Website set up by a medical institution or a clinical practice where patients and doctors can maintain two-way password protected communication and where access to an electronic health record enables the team to review medications, medical history, lab results, treatment programs, and other aspects of a patient's care.

Pay for Performance (P4P): A payment approach used in healthcare that correlates payment to a physician with how well the physician adheres to practice standards and achieves certain outcomes based on a set of performance measures.

Personal Digital Assistant (PDA): A handheld device that is a fully functioning computer able to access the Internet, send and receive email, take and receive images and photos, and can be used as a telephone, digital organizer, calendar, address book, notepad. The PDA enables the physician to access patient health records, prescribe medications, code and bill for procedures, and check on the latest information related to treatment of patients.

Personal Health Record: An electronic cumulative record of health-related information on an individual drawn from multiple sources that is created and managed by the individual. The integrity of the data in the ePHR and control of access to it are the responsibility of the individual (source: NAHIT).

PEW Internet and American Life Project: An initiative of the Pew Research Center, a nonprofit "fact tank" funded by the PEW charitable trusts founded by Joseph Pew. The PEW Internet and American Life Project provides information on the issues, attitudes, and trends shaping America and the world. Pew Internet explores the impact of the internet on children, families, communities, the work place, schools, health care, and civic/political life.

Primary Care Physician: A clinician who provides integrated healthcare services and who addresses a large majority of personal healthcare needs of patients in a sustained long-term relationship.

Privacy Rule: Legislation enacted by the U.S. Congress in 2003 to establish the first Federal privacy standards to protect patient health information.

Provider: Any registered health professional who administers care to a patient. This can also refer to healthcare delivery organizations.

Regional Health Information Organization (RHIO): A health information organization that brings together health care stakeholders within a defined geographic area and governs health information exchange among them for the purpose of improving health and care in that community (source: NAHIT).

Registries: Organized systems for the collection, storage, retrieval, analysis, and dissemination of information on individual persons to support health needs. This also includes government agencies and professional associations that define, develop, and support registries.

Radio Frequency Identification (RFID): Automatic identification based on radio waves, using devices called RFID tags or transponders, which include an integrated circuit for storing and processing information and an antenna for receiving and transmitting the signal. RFID is used in healthcare to match patients with medication and to track materials and people within the healthcare setting.

Robots: Mechanical devices that include the artificial intelligence to make them capable of performing a variety of complex tasks such as measuring blood pressure, heart rate, and body temperature, inspecting incisions and performing surgical tasks, monitored, and assisted by a physician.

Specialist: A healthcare provider who is trained in a specific area and offers care in that particular branch of medicine.

Smart Phones: Devices similar to a PDA that function as a phone, camera, and handheld computer and include access to the Internet, email, and can include an audio feature that enables the clinician to dictate notes into the device that can be transmitted to an electronic health record or stored and saved.

Telehealth: A broader definition of remote healthcare that is not specific to clinical services. Telehealth uses communication technology to provide care and incorporates videoconferencing, the transmission of images, and the use of patient portals, remote monitoring of vital signs, continuing medical education, and nursing call centers.

Telemedicine: The use of communication equipment to link healthcare practitioners and patients who are in different locations, allowing patients to receive care where and when it is needed.

Telerehabilitation: The clinical application of consultative preventative and therapeutics services via interactive telecommunication systems.

Virtual Reality (VR): Human–computer interface that simulates a realistic environment and allows users to interact with it.

Index